Marv —
Stay Strong!
M O'Hara

PROSTATE CANCER AND OTHER PROSTATE PROBLEMS:

PREVENTION & CURES

BY
OLYMPIAN MICHAEL O'HARA

Bookman LLC
Publishing & Marketing
www.bookmanmarketing.com

ISBN: 1-59453-224-9

Art Linkletter
8484 Wilshire Boulevard, Suite 205
Beverly Hills, California 90211

May 8, 2001

I have known and worked with Michael O'Hara during the past half-century, in a wide variety of endeavors. I never thought I'd be recommending his research work on such a startling subject as prostate cancer!

Like many other seniors, I have worried about getting this deadly disease, and, as President of the Center for Aging at UCLA, I have talked about it with some of the top doctors in the nation.

It is a puzzling, fatal, common cancer, and as Mike so clearly and simply states – "It is not a situation where 'one size fits all.'"

In this book, carefully and painstakingly researched, Mike has presented many options available to you, depending on your cancer "statistics" and your personal temperament.

This is must reading for every man who discovers (early, I hope) that he has prostate cancer.

Congratulations, Mike; this is a winner and far more important than all the International success you have had in the volleyball history of the Olympics.

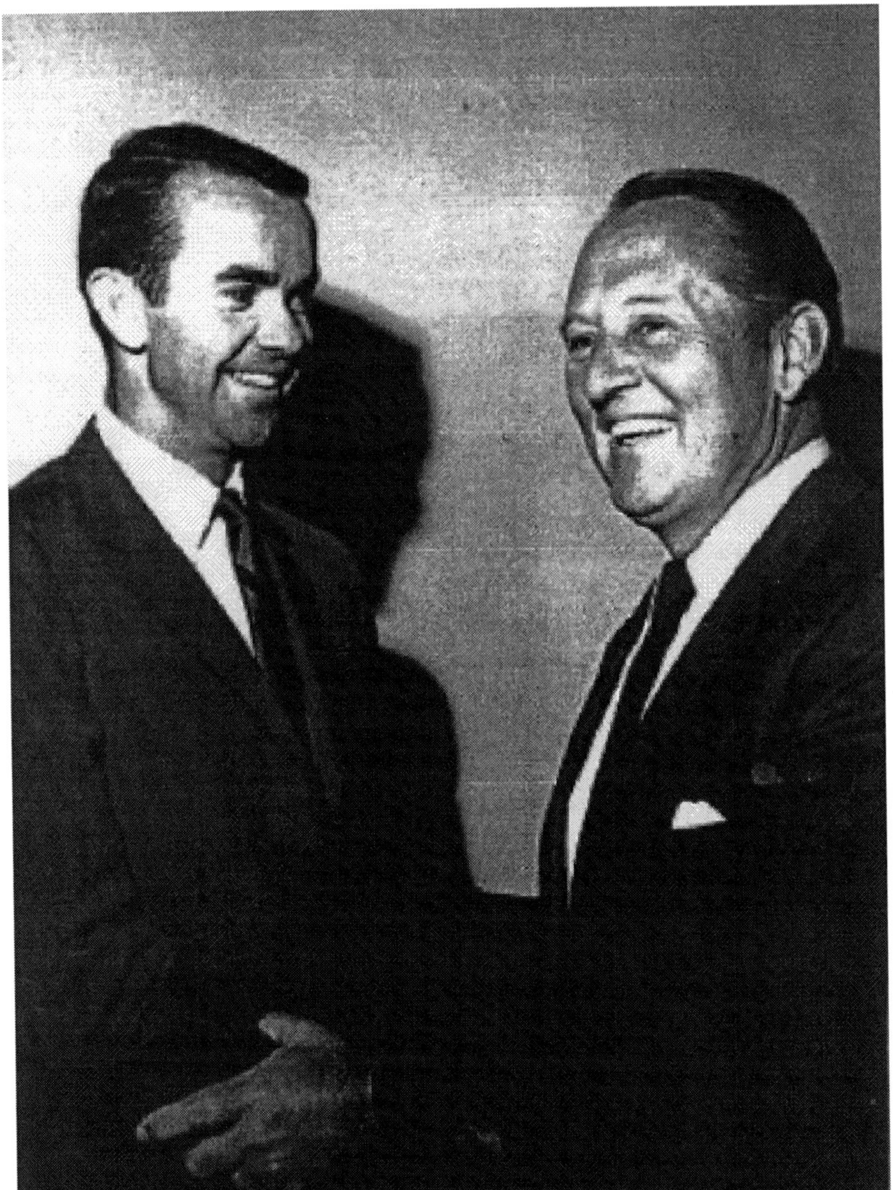

TABLE OF CONTENTS

PREFACE: Dr. John Blasko xi

SECTION I
WHY IT IS ESSENTIAL THAT PROSTATE CANCER PATIENTS BECOME EDUCATED QUICKLY AND IN DEPTH 1

Chapter 1
"Overview Of The Major Health Challenges Faced By Men" 3
Michael O'Hara, Olympian, College Business Instructor, Pacific Palisades. CA

Chapter 2
"The Shock Of My Life" 7
Michael O'Hara, Pacific Palisades, CA

Chapter 3
"Prostate Cancer Victim Michael O'Hara's Battle With The Forces Of Bias" 11
Michael O'Hara, Pacific Palisades, CA

Chapter 4
"The Role Played By HMO's Concerning Prostate Cancer Treatment" 33
Michael O'Hara, Pacific Palisades, CA

SECTION II
EXPERTS ANALYZE THE LATEST FACTS ABOUT PROSTATE CANCER PREVENTION AND TREATMENT CHOICES 37

Chapter 5
"Prostate Cancer Prevention Insights" 39
Dr. Charles "Snuffy" Myers, Founder and Medical Director, The American Institute for Diseases of the Prostate, Charlottesville, VA

Chapter 6
"Diet And Prostate Cancer" 59
from Dr. Mark Moyad, National Expert on Prostate Cancer Prevention, by Michael O'Hara

Chapter 7
"Radical Prostatectomy; Managing Localized Prostate Cancer" 69
Dr. Stanley Brosman, Santa Monica/UCLA Medical Center, CA

Chapter 8
"Radiation Therapy in the Management of Prostate Cancer" 83
Dr. Chris Rose, Chairman, American Society of Therapeutic Radiology and Oncology, Valley Radial Therapy Associates, Providence St. Joseph's Medical Center, Burbank, CA

Chapter 9
"Permanent Seed Implantation for Early Stage Prostate Cancer" 97
Dr. Peter Grimm, Chairman National Seeds Quality Assurance, Seattle Prostate Institute, WA

Chapter 10
"High Dose Rate Interstitial Implant (The Most Conformal of All)" 133
Physician Michael Steinberg, Radiation Oncologist, Santa Monica/UCLA Medical Center, CA

Chapter 11
"Intensity Modulated Radiation Therapy "IMRT" The New-New Thing" 141
Physician Michael Steinberg, Radiation Oncologist, Santa Monica/UCLA Medical Center, CA

Chapter 12
"Cyrosurgery Of The Prostate" 151
Dr. Stuart Fisher, UCLA School of Medicine, Past President - Society of Urological Cryosurgeons, Santa Monica, CA

Chapter 13
"Early Hormone Blockade In Men Suitable For Local Therapy" 159
Dr. Mark Scholz and Dr. Richard Lam, Hormone Therapy/ Oncology Specialists, Healing Touch Oncology - Marina del Rey, CA

Chapter 14
"New Approaches To Prostate Cancer Treatment" 171
Dr. Mark Scholz and Dr. Richard Lam, Hormone Therapy/Oncology Specialists, Healing Touch Oncology - Marina del Rey, CA

Chapter 15
"What's Wrong With The Watchful Waiting Posture That Is So Popular In Europe?" 183
Thomas Alexander, formerly Fortune Magazine science writer, "Oscar" winning article "One Man's Tough Choices On Prostate Cancer," Imaggie Valley, NC

Chapter 16
"Preventing And Curing Cancer By Working Through The Mind" 205
Dr. Al Barrios, Recipient of First Annual Cancer Federation Award, Psychoneuroimmunology and author of *Toward Greater Freedom and Happiness*, Los Angeles, CA

Chapter 17
"The Benefits Of Community Based Cancer Support Programs-Using The Wellness Community As An Example" 215
Dr. Harold Benjamin, Author of The Wellness Community Guide to Fighting for Recovery From Cancer, Wellness Community of Santa Monica, CA

SECTION III
REAL EXPERIENCES FROM REAL PEOPLE 221

Chapter 18
"Prostate Problems Aren't Always About Cancer" 223
Bill Toomey, Gold Medal Winning Olympic Decathlete

Chapter 19
"One Man's Burning, But Benign, Progress With His Prostate" . 229
Don Regan, Attorney/Co-Founder of American Basketball Association and World Hockey Association

Chapter 20
"Observations Regarding Radical Prostate Surgery" 237
Dick Archer, Insurance Executive, Santa Barbara, CA

Chapter 21
"My Prostate Cancer Shock" 255
Jack Schumacher, Insurance Executive, Brentwood, CA

Chapter 22
"There Is No They" 263
William K. Weinstein, Businessman, San Francisco, CA

Chapter 23
"Taking On Prostate Cancer" 313
Andy Grove, Ph.D., Intel Chairman, Santa Clara, CA

Chapter 24
"The Mountain Man Goes For Cryosurgery" 337

Chapter 25
"The Guardian Angel" 345
Arlen O'Hara, Homemaker, Pacific Palisades, CA

Chapter 26
"Hope For The Future" 349
Michael O'Hara, Pacific Palisades, CA

PREFACE

John C. Blasko, MD
Seattle Prostate Institute
Seattle, WA

Men diagnosed with prostate cancer face a bewildering array of treatment choices and enter a world of astonishingly contentious claims and counter claims from respected medical professionals. Family and loved ones who only want the best for their men find themselves confused and often angry because of conflicting medical advice. For readers of this book who bear the burden of recent diagnosis and their families trying to help, the pages that follow provide invaluable information about many of the advances in prostate cancer treatment available today. However, this book goes beyond the recitation of technical and medical description and offers insightful vignettes by articulate and perceptive men who describe their own journey through the maze of information about prostate cancer and how they reached a decision for their particular treatment. These chapters should be required reading for all physicians who counsel patients about prostate cancer, and will be reassuring to patients who are just beginning their search and find themselves frustrated because of conflicting information or unsympathetic, dogmatic physicians.

How is it that things have reached this state of disagreement and disarray? Why is it that so many physicians seem to be unfamiliar with new treatment approaches or dismiss them out of hand? Is it any wonder that patients lose confidence in their physicians and feel that they themselves must become expert in this disease? To understand why we have come to this state of affairs, we need to turn back the clock twenty years. In my medical training in the 1970s and my early years of practice as a radiation oncologist in the 1980s, prostate cancer treatment was relatively simple. There was surgery in the form of radical Prostatectomy, there was radiation in the form of external beam radiotherapy, and if you had cancer spread outside of the prostate you got a crude form of hormone therapy. Both urologists and radiation oncologists were smug in their belief that these treatments were highly effective and desirable. Debates about the merits of one versus the other were limited to mild skirmishes at local Tumor Boards but in the end, young patients with early cancers usually got surgery, older patients with more advanced cancers got external beam radiation and that's all there was to it. The first thing that shook this complacent world was the development of our friend the prostate specific antigen (PSA) blood test in the late 1980s. PSA is usually thought of as a test for the detection of prostate cancer but it is also a magnificent monitor of treatment success. When this sensitive new tool was applied to patients who had undergone either standard surgery or radiotherapy, we were shocked to find that neither surgery nor radiotherapy cured nearly as many patients as we had thought. To add insult to injury, there was a dawning awareness through quality of life studies that the impact on urinary, bowel, and sexual function from both surgery and radiation were profound and much greater than had been previously understood. To make matters even worse, data from Europe indicated that there were some patients with slow growing prostate cancers that didn't seem to need any treatment at all. Thus, the picture that emerged was that prostate cancer treatment rarely cured anybody but it sure did a lot of damage and maybe wasn't even necessary. What a turn of events in a few short years! Thus goaded, urologists, radiation oncologists, and recently medical oncologists went back to the drawing boards. The goal: for those patients who needed treatment, how could cure rates be improved while minimizing complications?

In the surgical world, physicians such as Patrick Walsh, MD at Johns Hopkins University and others developed nerve sparing techniques, greater understanding of prostate anatomy, and new techniques of controlling blood loss and sphincter preservation. These advances did breathe new life into an old procedure but surgery is fundamentally limited as a single dimension approach and can not take advantage of our imperfect but growing knowledge of cancer on the cellular level. For some cancer situations, however, it can be the best choice.

In the world of radiation treatments, the past 15 years has seen an explosion of technology that has led to multiple new approaches. A fundamental principle of radiation therapy is that the larger the cancer, the higher the dose of radiation needed to eradicate it. What we now realize is that the radiation doses we were capable of delivering 20 years ago were inadequate to completely destroy most prostate cancers. Thus, today's approaches are designed to either deliver higher doses to the prostate while minimizing radiation to the surrounding normal organs or manipulate the cancer environment so that a given dose of radiation is more effective. The technological breakthroughs that have enabled us to achieve these goals can be summarized as:

1. The development of prostate imaging tools such as transrectal ultrasound, CT scanning, and magnetic resonance imaging.
2. The medical applications of powerful computers to plan, control, and document the accurate delivery of radiation.
3. The recognition that hormone therapy is synergistic with radiation and can increase its effectiveness in certain cases.

These advances are translated into the current treatments of Brachytherapy (seed implants or high dose rate), 3-D conformal external beam radiotherapy, and the simultaneous use of androgen deprivation (hormone therapy) with either Brachytherapy or external beam. Excellent results at 10 years and beyond are now available for these new approaches accounting for their growing popularity. The chapters that follow provide a clear and accurate review for each of these new treatment approaches.

In the world of medical therapy, we have made great strides in developing more effective and better tolerated forms of hormone therapy and are beginning to take advantage of the synergism that exists with combinations of medical therapy and radiation. The distant future is very bright with promising work on genetic manipulation and vaccine treatments.

Consider the physician trained in the 1970s and 80s who had no exposure to these new treatments and the fact that most of the innovations came from outside the realm of urology. From these physicians perspective, change has come with the speed and terror of an avalanche. Caught flat-footed, immersed in busy practices, they find it difficult to assimilate and understand these new technologies much less master them. It is much easier to stick with the old. A further difficulty in accepting new treatments lies in the fact that they are all essentially evolutions of older techniques that used cruder technology and did not work particularly well. For example, seed implants were tried in the 60s by manually inserting needles into the prostate during an operation without any guidance system. The results with that approach were poor and so, when some physicians hear about seed implants today, their response is, "It didn't work before, why should it work now?" This ignores, of course, the fact that technology CAN improve things. Now that results are available to 10 years and beyond, it is clear that these new treatments do work and are assuming an increasing role in the management of patients with prostate cancer. Unfortunately, through ignorance, complacency, self-interest, or just laziness, there continue to be physicians who are either unfamiliar with new treatments or vociferously reject them in spite of the data. You will recognize physicians of this stripe as you read the personnel experiences in this book. Fortunately, they are becoming rarer.

No discussion of the rise in popularity of these treatments would be complete without mention of the invaluable role of the Internet. The Internet has proved to be a marvelous source of information and, unfortunately, misinformation. Many thousands of people have gained meaningful information about treatment choices through the Internet. When we were first developing seed implants in the late 1980s, the Internet was also beginning. In those early days of Brachytherapy we were being called lunatics and worse by many in the medical establishment. It was our early patients who were ecstatic about the results of their seed implant, that took to the Internet to provide an "underground" resource for others. Even today, many patients first learn of the seed implant treatment option through the Internet. It's a great resource - use it, but be alert for unreasonable claims.

Today, prostate cancer treatment is best viewed as individualized options rather than a "one size fits all" approach. Complicated and confusing? Yes, but in the end a better solution for you. So, how do you decide which treatment option is best for you? First, become educated so that you understand the basics of prostate cancer and learn the lingo of the disease. This does not mean you have to become a physician, but learn enough so that you know what questions to ask and can recognize a knowledgeable and open-minded physician from one who is not. Reading this book will go a long way in educating you. Second, find a physician who is knowledgeable and open to a variety of treatments and will spend the time necessary to answer your questions. Sometimes, for a variety of medical reasons, it may be that a single treatment is clearly best for a patient. More often there are several treatments that would be appropriate and you will have to decide which is best for you. This is a difficult decision because your life is on the line. Often this decision is part "head" and part "heart". The head part is your due diligence. Are the numbers right for your disease; is the outcome likely to be good? The heart part is your gut instinct as to which treatment you have the most confidence in. Which one feels "right" for you? In the end, only you can provide the answer.

FOREWORD

It was only a few years after the first moon landing in 1969 that cancer first affected my family and I began to focus on medical research. Back then, there was a lot of optimism. It seemed clear that if we could reach the moon we could find curses for serious diseases. Yet two decades later, millions more Americans, including my father, had died from cancer and we weren't much closer to a cure. Building on the earlier work of the Milken Family Foundation against several diseases, I established CaP CURE – the Association for the Cure of Cancer of the Prostate – in 1993 to jumpstart prostate cancer research. Since then, we've raised $160 million for research, including more than 80 human clinical trials of promising new treatments, and become the largest non-governmental source of funds for this vital work.

One out of every five men in America will be affected by prostate cancer in his lifetime. It's a very serious disease. That's the bad news. The good news is that we are making solid progress from the 43,000 men who died from this disease in the U.S. in 2000. This year only 30,000 will die. That number of deaths was expected to rise as increasing numbers of baby boomers reached the age at which prostate cancer is more likely to be diagnosed. Yet by 2001, remarkably, the number of prostate cancer deaths had declined to 31,500. While that is still a tragically large number, the 28% decline in deaths over eight years indicates that programs like those of CaP CURE are having a positive effect.

Another sign of progress is growing awareness. A decade ago, prostate cancer, like breast cancer a generation earlier, was "in the closet," something men didn't talk about. Now, men like Michael O'Hara *are* talking, and delivering information that will help save lives. Most men have at least heard about the PSA test, although not enough men ask their doctors for it. But the word is spreading. Tell your friends how important it is to get tested, to eat a healthy diet, and to support those organizations that are hot on the trail of a cure.

Michael Milken
Founder and Chairman, CaP CURE

ACKNOWLEDGEMENTS

THERE ARE MANY PEOPLE THAT HAVE MADE MAJOR CONTRIBUTIONS TO THIS BOOK. I MUST START WITH MY WIFE OF OVER FORTY YEARS, ARLEN, WHO JUMPED INTO THIS ADVENTURE WITH ME, AND HELPED ME DIGEST THE TWO DOZEN MEDICAL INTERVIEWS WITH SOME OF THE FINEST PHYSICIANS IN THE PROSTATE CANCER FIELD AND CONTRIBUTED HER EXCELLENT COMPUTER SKILLS. MY NEXT LINE OF DEFENSE WAS SON RYAN, DAUGHTER-IN-LAW VICTORIA AND HER SANTA MONICA LIBRARIAN MOTHER, BETSY, HELPING ME DO THE VITAL TWO MONTHS OF RESEARCH THAT LED TO MY PERSONAL DECISION REGARDING TREATMENT.

THE SUPPORT AND ASSISTANCE GIVEN ME THROUGHOUT, MY RESEARCH PERIOD BY MY DAUGHTER KELLEY, HER HUSBAND BILL PYETT, AND MY CREATIVE GRANDSON, SPENCER, WAS EQUALLY FABULOUS. OLD FRIENDS LUCILE AND JIM CAYTON ADDED SUPERB SUPPORT AND INCOURAGEMENT.

I MUST THANK MY OLD OLYMPIC GOLD MEDAL WINNING SWIMMER COMPATRIOT, JOHN NABOR, WHOSE LATEST PUBLICATION - “AWAKEN THE OLYMPIAN WITHIN” GAVE ME THE IDEA TO INVITE BOTH PHYSICIANS AND PROSTATE CANCER PATIENTS TO SHARE BOTH THE PAIN AND HONOR OF GIVING BIRTH TO THIS BOOK. THE WILLINGNESS TO SHARE THEIR PERSONAL EXPERIENCES, SUPPLIED BY THE “CREME DE LA CREME” OF THE MEDICAL PROFESSION, ALONG WITH THE MOST DIVERSE SYMPTOMS, TREATMENTS AND RESULTS OF THE FIFTY PLUS PALS THAT I INTERVIEWED IN ORDER TO MAKE THE RIGHT SELECTION FOR ME, CONTRIBUTED THE INGREDIENTS THAT UNQUESTIONABLY IS WHAT GIVES

THIS BOOK STRONG LEGS. THAT IS ESPECIALLY TRUE WITH THE ADDITION OF TWO OLYMPIC GOLD MEDAL WINNERS, BILL TOOMEY AND DOUG BEAL TO THE TEAM. TWO NEW PHYSICIANS, MARK MOYAD AND "SNUFFY" MYERS, WORLD CLASS SPECIALISTS IN PROSTATE CANCER PREVENTITIVE ACTIONS ALSO CONTRIBUTED MIGHTILY.

MY SPECIAL THANKS GO TO DR. MARK SCHOLZ AND GLENN WEAVER, CO-FOUNDER AND EXECUTIVE DIRECTOR RESPECTIVELY, OF PROSTATE CANCER RESEARCH INSTITUTE (PCRI), WHO SAW ONE OF MY PRESENTATIONS AND INVITED ME TO JOIN THEM IN THIS FIGHT TO AVOID DEATH BY CANCER. THAT ACTION ENABLED MY FRIENDS BOB WALLER, MERLE BANTA, JACK SCHUMACHER AND DICK ARCHER, FELLOW PROSTATE CANCER SUFFERERS, TO JOIN IN BY CONTRIBUTING FUNDS TO "PCRI-O'HARA FUND" (501C3), SUPPLYING SOME OF THE TRAVELING EXPENSES FOR OUR NATIONAL THRUST.

IT WAS A GREAT JOY TO HAVE MY OLD BOSS, ART LINKLETTER AND HIS CAPABLE ADMINISTRATOR, LEE RAY, COME TO MY AID WITH HIS GENEROUS LETTER. MY WONDERFUL EDITOR WAS DR. DARLENE KLUKA, WHOM I HAVE ENJOYED OVER THE YEARS WHILE SERVING ON VARIOUS USAV BOARDS IN ORDER TO HELP OUR FAVORITE SPORT - VOLLEYBALL, CONTINUE TO GROW.

I WANT TO EXPRESS MY GRATITUDE TO MY TWO LONG TIME FRIENDS AND NEIGHBORS, TELEVISION AND PLAY AUTHORS, JIM MCGINN AND PETER NELSON WHO TAUGHT ME THAT BREVITY IS THE KEY TO WRITING PARADISE!

MY SURGEON, DR. PETER GRIMM, INTRODUCED ME TO HIS ASSOCIATE - DR. CHARLES HEANEY, AND THE THREE OF US HAVE HAD GREAT FUN "GROWING" THIS BOOK EVER SINCE. THEY, IN TURN, HELPED ME INVITE THEIR WORLD

RENOWN SPECIALIST IN THIS FIELD, DR. JOHN BLASKO, TO CONTRIBUTE THE PREFACE TO THIS PUBLICATION.

MY SPECIAL THANKS TO BOB GAIRDNER, AN OLD FRIEND AND PROSTATE FRATERNITY BROTHER, WHO WAS THE FIRST PERSON TO RECOMMEND DR. PETER GRIMM, WHO WAS HIS PHYSICIAN FOR THE SEED IMPLANTATION PROCEDURE. THANKS ALSO TO MY SMC BUSINESS STUDENTS JEANENE BENTLEY AND ELLEN FLOYD FOR THEIR EDITING ASSISTANCE.

MANY THANKS FOR A TERRIFIC COVER DESIGN GENEROUSLY DONATED BY RENOWNED CANADIAN DESIGNER JOHN BAYER.

FINALLY, I WANT TO EXPRESS MY GRATITUDE TO ROTARY DISTRICT GOVERNOR INGO WERK, A FELLOW PROSTATE CANCER VICTIM, WHO HAS JOINED OUR ADVISORY COMMITTEE IN THIS BATTLE ON A WORLDWIDE BASIS. OUR OTHER TALENTED MEMBERS ARE JOHN LEHNE, DON MELLIG, CONNOLLY OYLER, DR. DAVID ROGERS, LIONEL RUHMAN, AND DR. MARK SCHOLZ.

Healthy mind, Healthy Body. Professor O'Hara exemplifies the title Olympian in his passion for life. *Prostate Cancer and Other Prostate Problems: Prevention & Cures* serves to show society how we can all live better and longer in pursuit of excellence. Higher, Swifter, Stronger...a motto which will guide you through this book.

Liston Bouchette
Secretary General
World Olympians Association

The World Olympians Association is a global organization dedicated to unifying Olympians for fraternal benefits and community service. From time to time the WOA promotes the efforts made by Olympians in a non-profit function aimed to support public welfare.

INTRODUCTION

When I decided to update my first book "Prostate Cancer Battle: It's Strictly Your Decision", I felt that it was imperative that I expand it to include several additional issues. In my speeches, and television and radio interviews, over the last two years on this subject, I did just that. I found that my most provocative speech title was "The Inside Scoop on the Olympic and Prostate Cancer Fraternities!" First, I discussed the fraternity that everyone wanted to be in – the Olympic Movement, and then the one that NO ONE wanted to be in, Prostate Cancer! But in many cases, it's compulsory! The questions addressed to me came back loud and clear: How do I, or someone I love, avoid contracting this killer disease in the first place?" I was amazed at the number of women who had a dad, brother or husband that they wanted to protect and educate.

The second most frequently asked question was "what about the other problems concerning the prostate, other then Cancer?" My research into this subject nearly floored me! OVER 50% OF THE MEN IN THE WORLD WILL SUFFER FROM PROSTATE PROBLEMS, AND HALF OF THOSE WILL CONTRACT CANCER. That means that approximentally 1.75 billion men will face prostate problems!

That meant, in addition to appealing to the terrific team of Doctors that I invited to help me with the first book to respond to these two vital questions, I had to have them refer me to physicians that specialize in those two specific areas. Two of the world leaders in this field, Doctors Charles "Snuffy" Myers and Mark Moyad, have joined me in this effort. I am tremendously pleased with the information that is contained in this missive, concerning those topics, as the result of those generous contributions.

SECTION I

WHY IT IS ESSENTIAL THAT PROSTATE CANCER PATIENTS BECOME EDUCATED QUICKLY AND IN DEPTH

Chapter 1

"OVERVIEW OF THE MAJOR HEALTH CHALLENGES FACED BY MEN"

by Michael O'Hara

There are four major diseases that are KILLERS OF MAN. Therefore, PREVENTION and CURES are the life saving messages to give each man, some three billion throughout the world, to afford those individuals the best possible chance for survival. The four major killers are HEART ATTACKS, LUNG CANCER, COLON CANCER AND PROSTATE CANCER.

We now have coronary scanning devices that will identify whether your heart is building up the excessive plaque that causes it to break down. This checkup should be done, starting at fifty, every three years. Once a problem is identified, happily there are effective pills to reduce the plaque, and keep your heart healthy. Pfizer sells six billion dollars a year worth of Lipitor, while less popular but effective is the newest prescription drug on the market, Zetia, along with over-the-counter products - Niacin and Folic Acid. (Note: see your doctor before deciding which is right for you).

If you don't smoke, the percentage of men with Lung Cancer problems becomes infinitesimal. Tragically, while seventy percent of all smokers want to stop, the quit rate of those who try to break their nicotine addiction ranges between five and eight percent.

Colon Cancer is the second biggest killer of the four, (behind Lung Cancer), with over 147,000 cases a year, in the U.S. alone, for which there is no hormone blocking safety net. The good news is that the detection test is very effective. Everyone, from the age of fifty on, should have a colonoscopy every five years. However, be sure you discuss any negative family history with your physician, since it may mandate your starting checkups at an earlier age. Any small polyps will be removed during the process and, only if a major problem arises, will a more serious procedure be needed. Genetech has a new drug being tested by the Food and Drug Administration, called Avastin, that is reputed to be the answer for those extreme cases.

The fourth and last of the major Man Killers is Prostate Cancer, from which no one dies directly. However, if the Cancer is virulent, and if it escapes the shell, then you will die, since it will ultimately infect some of your vital organs, (stomach, liver, brain, etc). The latest statistics are increasingly scary. ONE HALF OF ALL MEN WILL HAVE PROSTATE PROBLEMS, AND FIFTY PERCENT OF THOSE PROBLEMS WILL BE CANCER!

The major non Cancer problem is called "Benign Prostate Hyperplasia" or BPH. By the age of fifty, 33% of males will have problems urinating, caused by prostate growth. Some recent research statistics indicate that almost ALL men will have Prostate problems some time in their life. That is why it is important that we also discuss the other prostate problems, in addition to Cancer, as well as preventative measures for both. Once again, smoking, obesity and high fat diets increase the likelihood of having this embarrassing problem. Since these same factors negatively impact all four of the above Man Killers, a disciplined approach is called for. This BPH condition accounts for 375,000 hospital stays per year in the United States.

For that reason, when dealing with the prostate, it is important to discuss both Cancer and non Cancer concerns, as well as preventative measures for both conditions.

The good news is that all four of these Man Killers can be defeated, or deferred, if you learn the optimum preventative steps to adopt, and take action!

The best attack on all four of these man killers is taking responsibility for your own health. These medicines and tests are available to deal with the specific problem, in many cases preventatively, or at least postponed it by keeping fit and eating the right foods. Amazingly, many people take care of their car better than they do their own bodies! The key words are "cardio vascular" and "strength training". The stronger you are, the longer you live!

So the initial hurdle is ignorance, and it can only be overcome by education. It is vital that you keep an inquiring mind - when you stop learning, you start dying. This process is not a photograph, it is a motion picture. You must continually keep up with the latest discoveries in the health field.

For me, my experience in a high school chemistry lab paid off in more then just receiving a good grade. Mrs. Redlands, at Santa Monica High School, had each student take a coin and examine it under a microscope. She then produced several quart bottles of Coke, gave each student a glass for the coke, and we left each coin in "our" glass overnight. The next morning, the microscope depicted each damaged coin, and I have never had a Coke, or any other cola since!

Even more importantly, the following month she also took us on a field trip to the Santa Monica morgue, where the class was able to examine two corpses, one eaten brutally with lung cancer and one that had not smoked. That comparative experience completely removed any temptation for me to smoke for the rest of my life.

Therefore, when I decided to update my first book "Prostate Cancer Battle: It's Strictly Your Decision", I felt that it was imperative that I expand it to include these crucial additional issues. In my speeches, and television and radio interviews, over the last two years on this subject, I did some marketing research, regarding what my various audiences really wanted to know. For example, I found that the most provocative speech title was "The Inside Scoop on the Olympic and Prostate Cancer Fraternities!" First, I discussed the fraternity that everyone wanted to be in - the Olympic Games, and then the one that NO ONE wanted to be in, Prostate Cancer! Many times, the speech chairman would invite me for the Olympic subject, because of it's affirmative values, but wind up thanking me for the Prostate Cancer update. In some cases, weeks later I sometimes received notes indicating that some of their members lives had been saved! That was every bit as gratifying as a note from a former college student attributing some business success to what he or she learned in my classroom.

The constant query came back loud and clear: "How do I, or someone I love, avoid contracting this killer disease in the first place?" I was amazed at the number of women who had a dad, brother or husband that they wanted to educate and protect.

The second most frequently asked question was "what about the problems concerning the prostate, other then Cancer?" My research into this subject nearly floored me! Since well over half the men in the world will be effected, sometime in their life, that means that over two billion men will face prostate problems!

I immediately appealed to the terrific team of doctors that I invited to participate with me in the first book, in addition to updating their chapters, to respond to these two additional questions. I also had them identify the best physicians that specialize in those two specific areas. I am pleased with the information that is contained in this missive concerning those vital elements, as the result of their generous and thoughtful contributions.

I then persuaded several Gold Medal Olympic champions, Bill Toomey and Doug Beal, to lead the charge in illuminating the current challenge of dealing with this embarrassing and omnipresent condition called BPH, from a patient's point of view. They have answered the call in the same masterful way in which they dealt with their sport, decathlon and volleyball respectively.

Chapter 2

THE SHOCK OF MY LIFE

by Michael O'Hara

"Michael, you have prostate cancer." My physician continued to speak...but I was too shocked to hear what he said. I was convinced that my life was over. How long did I have? Weeks? Months? A year?

I staggered out of his office, drove home to tell my wife, Arlen, and, with her encouragement, started the most important research project of my life. This book is the result of that research. Prostate Cancer is the most common cancer in America, second only to lung disease, as the most common cause of death. It has been diagnosed much more frequently since screening by a new blood test, Prostate Specific Antigen (PSA) was introduced in 1988. Twenty-five percent of men in their 30's have microscopic prostate cancer. In their 50's the percentage rises to forty percent. Some of those cancer cells remain dormant, but some grow and expand ultimately beyond the prostate shell.

Early in my business career, I was fortunate to be hired as a trouble shooter by television host Art Linkletter. Art had several distressed multi-million dollar business ventures. One was in Arizona, a collection of motels, a rental complex and private airport, suffering during the mid-60's when Arizona was over built. Another was a large Southern California retirement development. In analyzing these and other new business opportunities for Art, I learned to perform "due diligence" before formulating a recommendation with strength and conviction. This patient, objective approach has served me well throughout my business career.

I took the same approach in dealing with my Prostate Cancer dilemma. I developed a two month timetable to research every aspect of this life threatening subject. I utilized the Internet, libraries, book stores, professional specialists, friends and other contacts who had faced a similar challenge and were willing to share the extremely sensitive details with me.

I was very frustrated by the lack of published information that could aid my research. Eighty percent of the current articles and books were written by physicians for physicians. I have an MBA and have been a college business professor for four decades years, but this was harder to understand than the legalese written by and for lawyers. The myriad of technical terms, charts, and diagrams used were impossible to comprehend. One physician explained to me that he would never "dumb down" a written presentation just to make it understandable for cancer patients.

The other twenty percent of the written information was anecdotal in nature from an individual patient who had enjoyed success with a particular treatment. The key question is, what success would be achieved by the next 100 men using that same technique. Also, since the writer's medical "statistics" are customized to that individual, they may not apply to many of the readers.

I made a plan to identify and access several dozen prostate cancer specialists throughout America that were the best and the brightest. I found most of them to be extremely knowledgeable, as well as very skilled, persuasive Marketeers. This was especially true when I began to expand my interviews beyond the medical professionals in my HMO. (Note: Due to the importance of that subject I have described my HMO experience in more detail in Chapter 4)

During that series of interviews of star medical professionals in each of the pertinent prostate cancer disciplines, a major change occurred in me. For the first time in my sixty-seven years, the pedestal upon which I had always placed all physicians was destroyed. I came to learn that, when your life is on the line, that pedestal can cost you your lifestyle or even cause your death.

The eight medical professionals who share their knowledge in this reader-friendly compendium are those whom I felt were the most expert in their specific prostate cancer specialty. These super star physicians are also the ones that I felt to be the most fair in their presentation of ALL of my alternative treatment options.

The seven patient case studies I have presented are a cross section of different prostate cancer statistics, treatment decisions, and results. This enables the reader to match up his own prostate cancer measurements to whichever case study he most closely approximates. My collaborators are both old friends and new, who want to help the next person thrust into this unique fraternity. This book is also an excellent tool for loved ones who want to learn what this formidable opponent to a happy lifestyle is all about.

After nine weeks of intensive research and many contradictions and frustrations, I selected the treatment option that fit my personal lifestyle and feelings the best. The decision that I made may not be the right one for you. This is definitely not a situation where "one size fits all." You must select from the many current options based upon your cancer "statistics" and your personal temperament.

Each of these physicians and friends join me in standing ready to help. You will find addresses and telephone numbers of many of them at the back of this publication. The frustration I suffered, especially from the lack of current, patient-friendly information, at a time for a crucial decision, strongly motivated me to write both of my books.

Chapter 3

PROSTATE CANCER VICTIM MICHAEL O'HARA'S BATTLE WITH THE FORCES OF BIAS

by Michael O'Hara

At the risk of coming up to the plate swinging very hard, let me immediately give you one of the first important punch lines of this book. When initially faced with the news that your biopsy test results indicate that you have prostate cancer, it is vital that you do not accept the first offer of medical help that you receive.

This initial sales pitch may be very hard to resist since it will usually be presented by an intelligent, extremely well-educated physician who strongly believes in what he is proposing. He is strongly motivated by his commitment to medicine, his intensive training in the field and, possibly, by the considerable monetary rewards that he will receive.

A periodic blood test measures the level of protein called Prostate-Specific Antigen (PSA). Prostate cancer can just be an indolent disease unlikely to cause lasting harm to your health. Its treatment, however, will usually cause serious side effects, like impotence and incontinence.

The surgical removal of a prostate will range in cost between \$20,000.00 to \$30,000.00. Additionally, the surgeon acquires a patient for life. Similar to the treatment of an alcoholic, the physician will frequently monitor your condition, administer periodic PSA tests and monitor all of the other sensitive and critical organs located in the same area, in addition to your prostate.

If the results of the surgery are extremely positive, your physician may even ask you to contribute a tax-deductible gift to his University or Foundation, thereby increasing his monetary rewards. At the very least you will be asked to be on his referral list to assist him in securing more prostate cancer patients. To add to the intrigue, even though he may touch briefly on some of the other treatment approaches available, every primary pitch tends to be that of recommending surgery.

One of the primary reasons for this recommendation is very basic. When the blood test part of your periodic physical examination indicates that your PSA has started to climb, your internist or general practitioner will refer you to a urologist. When the urologist informs you that your prostate biopsy reveals that you have cancer, most patients are placed in the most vulnerable position possible. It is at this point that, in my opinion, one of the greatest travesties in medicine occurs. There are over 8500 urologists in the United States and <u>every one of them is a surgeon</u>...it's like choosing to become religious and going to a Catholic Priest and asking him which religion you should select. Unless you schedule meetings with a Rabbi and a Minister as well, you're going to be presented with a biased picture from which to make your religious decision and you'll probably end up a Catholic.

Two conditions make the prostate cancer decision an unfair environment for the new patient. First, most of us have been conditioned from childhood to respect and follow the medical advice from the physicians that our parents selected for us. Second, when initially informed that you have failed your biopsy and you have cancer, concerns about your mortality tend to place you almost under the complete control of your urologist.

The surgical operation itself is a highly sensitive one. The walnut sized prostate is positioned directly below the bladder. The urethra, which handles your urine flow, runs through it. Most importantly, the prostate is responsible for delivering your ejaculate. When you start dealing with potency and continence, you are involving the essence of masculinity. Just to make the neighborhood even more sensitive, the anus is only a few millimeters away and the testicles are right next door.

Surgeons love the challenge of performing this delicate operation. When a surgery is successful, it's a tremendous "high" for the surgeon, as well as a considerable relief for the patient. Since many of the classical surgical operations have been replaced by radiation treatment, the prostate operation is one of the "Last of the Mohicans." Even breast cancer treatments involve more alternatives than just the removal of the breast. Ten years ago, breast removal was almost automatically determined to be the primary treatment. It is now considered somewhat barbaric. In five more years, the same may be true for prostate surgery. The challenge of any of the available treatments is to eradicate the cancer cells in and on the periphery of the prostate without injuring any of the contiguous healthy and highly sensitive organs.

Time constraints become another huge consideration. While Prostate Cancer is considered to be a relatively slow growing cancer, there is no way to identify whether specific cancer cells are passive or virulent. If they are passive, you could live the rest of your life "watchfully waiting." This approach consists of essentially eating the right foods, living a healthy lifestyle, and waiting to see how active your cancer cells become. That is what the vast number of European and Asian prostate cancer patients do. Unfortunately international physicians appear to be making the decision for their patients, advising them to not have periodic PSA tests, or failing to mention the PSA test availability at all. They consider Americans to be "cut and burn happy." History indicates that over 80% of the corpses analyzed for cancer have recorded cancer of the prostate, but usually one does not die from it. However as discoveries like the Genome identification system make greater longevity a reality, more will die from it.

Thus, if cancer cells escape from the prostate shell, because they are virulent, they will attack other organs such as the stomach, kidney, and brain. Death from the extension of prostate cancer becomes almost a certainty. Because it is not possible to clearly measure the growth potential of your specific type of prostate cancer cells, your urologist may try to motivate you to place yourself on his surgical procedure schedule immediately.

If you accept that invitation you are playing Russian Roulette... with a Russian! If you don't get second and third opinions from other reputable surgeons, as well as top flight external radiation physicians, then from internal radiation physicians, you are dealing with this crucial decision to your distinct disadvantage.

Additionally, you should immediately request your biopsy slides and report from your urologist. They should be sent to the analyzer of prostate cancer cells reputed to be the best in the world, Dr. John Epstein, Johns Hopkins Hospital, Baltimore, Maryland (see Figure 1) For just a few hundred dollars you can make sure that a crucial measurement of your Prostate Cancer condition has been accurately analyzed. According to my research, in many cases original analyses have been inaccurate.

When presented with a life threatening condition like prostate cancer, you owe it to your loved ones, as well as to yourself, to seek out several of the best specialists in each of the disciplines. This is also the ideal time to identify and meet with the best oncologists, who usually do not have a particular treatment to sell. These physicians can provide far more objective information regarding your situation. They can also identify the best physicians for you to contact. Their personal referral will usually assist you in securing an early appointment. The most unbiased of all the physicians that I interviewed was oncologist Mark Scholz of Marina del Rey, California. He became a tremendous knowledge source, identifying the finest specialists for each treatment. Equally important, they can also help you determine where the latest state of the art equipment is located. <u>ONLY THE COMBINATION OF THE BEST PHYSICIAN</u>

WITH THE BEST EQUIPMENT IN EACH DISCIPLINE SHOULD BE CONSIDERED.

My personal research revealed some astounding results. For example, many of or most surgical procedures do not use the all-important "nerve sparing procedure" that is responsible for preserving men's penile erections. More recent advances in the surgical technique nationally has improved this approach considerably, and will be explored in detail by Dr. Stanley Brosman in a later chapter. Also, approximately 90% of all external radiation treatments are administered to Prostate Cancer patients using less than the best equipment available in the marketplace. The skill and experience level regarding internal radiation - Brachytherapy ("Seeds") - appears to dip considerably when you go beyond the superb medical facilities available in Seattle and Tampa.

The oncologist can also more objectively advise you, based upon your PSA and biopsy statistics whether an immediate decision regarding treatment is essential for your specific situation. Obviously, the more time you have to do your research, the better your decision will be, and the better you will feel about that decision.

The first action step should be to design your timed plan of attack. Figure 2 describes a PERT Chart, which stands for Production Evaluation Review Technique. This chart was designed by the British military to systematically attack German submarines with aircrafts during WWII. It was imminently successful and has subsequently been adopted by aerospace and electronic firms throughout the United States for management purposes. This tool was essential in helping me to reach the correct treatment decision for my custom situation.

The mental approach to this condition is just as important as it has been proven to be with cancer of the brain, colon and breast (Chapter 17). The better you feel about your research and your ultimate decisions concerning treatment, the better your mind and body will be able to battle your cancer, leading to improved health and longevity.

Figure 3 is a list of aggressive questions that my wife and I developed, supplemented by Dr. Peter Grimm, in order to glean the optimum research information from each initial meeting with some two dozen prostate cancer specialists. I also created my own personal slogan, developed to secure a reaction from each physician that I interviewed, when I felt one was appropriate - "I don't care if you cut, burn, or freeze me as long as you assure me that you can cure me." I found it extremely effective in clearing the air regarding my lack of aversion to any of the available treatments. The best physicians at fielding these questions were physicians Stanley Brosman, Michael Steinberg, Chris Rose, Stuart Fisher and Peter Grimm, who have generously contributed chapters on their specialties in great detail in this book.

Figure 4 is typical of the type of report received when meeting with those prominent prostate cancer treatment physicians. Once I had assembled all of the available data, including copious notes taken by my wife and me at each medical session, I caught an airplane to Sydney, Australia. My friends on the Australian Olympic Committee, Olympic Organizing Committee, and International Olympic Committee were having some challenges with the 2000 Games starting September 15, 2000.

The ten days in Sydney and Honolulu, including thirty hours on an airplane, gave me a chance to objectively digest all of the research material and come to a reasoned decision. The industry data provided by Wessels, Arnold & Henderson, with additional contributions from Dr. Peter Grimm (Figure 5) helped me considerably in arriving at my decision. Figure 6 describes a decision making process that has served all of the members of the O'Hara family well for many years, whenever a major decision has been called for. The left hand side identifies the prostate cancer conditions I felt to be most important to me. I then rated each on a scale from one to ten in importance. Then each prostate cancer treatment was weighed against those vital conditions on the same scale, and multiplied by the rating number, yielding a valid, definitive conclusion.

The winning conclusion for me turned out to be Internal Radiation (Brachytherapy Seeds). Note that the 380 point score was only a few percentage points greater than the external radiation score of 363. This evaluation is all very subjective and personal. There is seldom any one bright and shining answer - just various shades of gray. Upon my return I immediately flew to Seattle and met with Dr. Peter Grimm of the Seattle Prostate Institute at the Swedish Medical Center (Figure 7). I asked him aggressive questions, which he fielded flawlessly, and we hit it off beautifully. His associate, John Blasko, is their "Dr. Outside," giving speeches nationwide. Grimm is "Dr. Inside," performing more and more of the Seeds implantation procedures. Both have done thousands of these procedures and are known by most experts to be the best in the world, along with Dr. Michael Dattoli of the Center for Cancer Care in Tampa, Florida. I had made an appointment to meet with Dr. Dattoli the following week after a terrific 70-minute telephone conversation with him. However my meeting with Dr. Grimm affirmed to me that he was the right medical partner for me and I canceled my meetings with Dr. Dattoli, as well as meetings with two prominent, world class surgeons, Dr. Donald Skinner of USC and Dr. Robert Smith of UCLA.

My Seeds implantation took place on January 27th, 2000, (Figure 8-Operative Report). I was given my choice of the type of Seeds that I wanted, choosing between iodine and palladium. Dr. Grimm informed me that Palladium Seeds were initially stronger in radiation but had a shorter life span. I immediately asked what he would choose if he was in my shoes. His recommendation for me was iodine because they best fit my medium range PSA count and because they were delivered in clusters rather than individual Seeds, affording him the ability to apply them more effectively. I opted for, and received, 138 Iodine Seeds (I-125) produced by Amagyn Medical Technologies, Inc. in Irvine, California. As with all of the sound advice given me by Dr. Grimm, this turned out to be an impeccable decision.

The implantation procedure took forty minutes and was far less uncomfortable than my original forty-minute biopsy, which felt like a large stapling gun was being fired into my privates, as eighteen strips of my prostate were removed for observation. I stayed in Seattle for a check up the next morning and attended several business meetings in Los Angeles the following day. The day after that was Sunday, so I played my usual three hour morning doubles tennis competition at Mountaingate Country Club.

One year after my seed implantation I received a follow up concerning research that Dr. Grimm and his team was conducting (Figure 9) on a key element in this field - urinary retention. Prostate Cancer Institute is a leading force in this evolving environment, striving to find the optimum solutions for their patients. This same trio of physicians have also been conducting seminars across the country for other prostate cancer physicians that want to be able to offer some of their patients their thirteen year old, affirmatively tested method of seed implantation procedure.

My strength and all around good health never deserted me before, during or after the Seeds implantation. Exactly three months later, I was given a blood test to measure my PSA. I was warned by my new terrific, unbiased local urologist from UCLA/Santa Monica Hospital, Dr. Stanley Brosman, that my PSA might stay in the 7's and 8's or possibly drop down to 6 or 5, since the radiation life of Iodine Seeds was 6 to 8 months, usually yielding reductions somewhat evenly along the way. Three days later his nurse, Maritsa, called with great news - my PSA reading was 1.61! (Figure 10). Subsequent ninety-day PSA readings have stayed in the 1.1 to 1.4 range. Since then my bi-annual PSA count has remained under 1.00 and I continue to feel great. (Figure 11).

As a payback for my good fortune, I decided to create this book to arm you as you "go to war." I sincerely hope that <u>your</u> research, decision making and treatment of prostate cancer, or any other prostate problem, be as successful as mine.

Figure 1

Dec. 16.99 10:19

THE JOHNS HOPKINS HOSPITAL SURGICAL PATHOLOGY

Patient: O'HARA. MICHAEL Path # 599-4197

Temp ID # 8864678 Accessioned 11/30/1999

Birthdate: 09/15/1932 (Age 67) Loc: OUTSIDE

Gender: M Spec. Taken 11/10/1999

Outside Physician: JUDY H. KO, M.D.

INTERPRETATION AND DIAGNOSIS: (jxs) 12/07/1999

PROSTATE (N. O.S.. W99-13079):

RIGHT (A1): SMALL FOCUS OF ADENOCARCINOMA OF THE PROSTATE, GLEASON GRADE 3+3=6 IVOLVING TWO CORES (10%, 5%) (BLACK INKED CORES). SEE NOTE.

A2): PROSTATE TISSUE WITH FOCUS OF BENIGN CROWDED GLANDS.

LEFT (B1): SMALL FOCUS OF ADENOCARCINOMA OF THE PROSTATE, GLEASON GRADE 3+3= INVOLVING TWO CORES (5%, 2%) (BLACK INKED CORES).
SEE NOTE.

B2): MINUTE FOCUS OF ADENOCARCINOMA OF THE PROSTATE, GLEASON GRADE 3+3= 6 (BLUE INKED CORE). SEE NOTE.

NOTE: The diagnosis of carcinoma is supported by the failure of immunoperoxidase staining for high molecular weight cytokeratin to demonstrai basal cells in the atypical glands.

JONATHAN I. EPSTEIN. M.D. JIE

GROSS DESCRIPTION

PART #1: OUTSIDE SLIDES (sxz)
Resident Pathologist: JOSEPH D. Kronz. M.D. 11/30/1999

This specimen consists of eighteen slides labeled W99-13079 from Kaiser Permanente Medical Center in Los Angeles, CA.

Figure 2

MOH PERT CHART

November '99	December '99	January 2000
Blood test PSA up 8.7 Biopsy (flunked)	Evaluation period Identify "stars"- surgery, seeds, 3D Conformal, IMRT, Cryosurgery	Develop aggressive questions for doctors. Meet w/ doctors Make decision and schedule treatment
Secure 2nd opinion on biopsy analysis	Schedule appoint- ments w/doctors Read all current articles and books on PC	Read articles and books on PC

February 2000	March 2000	April 2000
Have treatment	Diet	Take PSA blood test
Identify and use diet	Write book	Diet
Employ psychological boost	Seek publisher	

Figure 3

Chapter 3 Questionnaire

QUESTIONS TO ASK PROSTATE CANCER TREATMENT PHYSICIANS

1. What is the stage of my cancer? What is the likelihood that it has spread to the lymph nodes, to the seminal vesicles, through the capsule.

2. What is the likelihood that the cancer is outside the treatment field?

3. Do you feel that a second opinion on the biopsy specimen is indicated? Are you satisfied with the number of biopsies?

4. What is the Gleason score of my cancer?

5. Do I require further tests? Why or why not?

6. For Urologist: how many prostate cancer operations have you performed?
   For Radiation Oncologist: how many patients have you treated with Conformal EBRT or Seeds?

7. What treatment options are available to me? What are the advantages and disadvantages of each?

8. What are my treatment options, including "watchful waiting?" (Surveillance)

9. What data is available to support each treatment option? How relevant and how current is that data? Is it based upon the experience of the outstanding physician in that treatment category only?

10. What do you define as successful treatment, and why? (Absolute PSA, PSA progression, etc.)

11. What are the risks of complications from each treatment? What kinds of complications are likely from each treatment? How are the complications themselves treated, i.e. impotence or incontinence?

12. Does your Center perform conformal beam? (all conformal is 3-dimensional).

13. What can I do to improve my recovery in terms of exercise and diet?

14. If I choose the surgery, would the surgeon use nerve sparing techniques?

15. If I select external radiation would my physician have the most current equipment to apply 3-D Conformal treatment?

16. How much will exercising help after the treatment has been supplied? How much will diet play a part in recuperation and what specific foods should I eat and avoid?

17. How fast would any radioactivity from the various internal and external radiation treatments dissipate? Is that good?

18. Since Palladium dissipates its radiation energy more quickly, is there any proof that it is better than iodine (I-125) or vice versa?

19. Which urologist and radiation oncologist would you suggest is an expert in this treatment nationally and locally, as a person to give me another opinion, and why?

20. Could I have a list of your previous prostate cancer patients to talk with?

Figure 4

Saint John's Health Center
Department of Radiation Oncology
CONSULTATION REPORT

November 23, 1999
PT: OHARA, MICHAEL
MR# M0516409
CNC#: 99-367
PHYSICIAN: ROBERT C. WOLLMAN, MD
PRIMARY PHYSICIAN:
REFERRING PHYSICIAN:

DIAGNOSIS: Prostate cancer, T1c, PSA 6.65, Gleason score 6

CHIEF COMPLAINT: The patient is a 67-year-old male with prostate cancer, seen in radiation therapy consultation.

NARRATIVE: The patient is a 67-year-old male whose PSA history is as follows: In June 1998, 3.6; in September 1999, 8.89; in October 5, 1999, 6.65. Sextant biopsies were performed on November 10, 1999. Bilateral adenocarcinoma, Gleason score 3 + 3 = 6 was found in one of three cores from the left midgland, two of three cores from the left apex, and two of three cores from the right apex. Invasion was noted to be focal and less than 1 mm. The patient is collecting opinions.

IMPRESSION AND PLAN: The patient is a 67-year-old male with clinically localized prostate cancer. The patient, his wife, and I had a long discussion regarding the controversies with regard to the most appropriate management. The patient understands that there is no "correct" and inviolable treatment for a man in his situation. The literature contains no long-term nonbiased randomized clinical trials comparing various modes of therapy to each other or to watchful waiting. The patient understands that numerous guideline committees have outlined radical prostatectomy, radiation therapy, and watchful waiting/androgen deprivation, all as appropriate depending on the clinical situation. We discussed his cancer and its prognostic features as well as its likelihood of having spread per the Partin tables. We discussed the various forms of radiation therapy (external beam, conformal external beam, radioactive implant, either alone or combined with external beam, and any of the above, combined with androgen deprivation). All of the side effects and the way each of the treatments are performed were detailed. We went over a four-step strategy for decision-making, primarily based on understanding the cancer, understanding the treatments, and understanding the patient.

All of the patient's and his wife's questions were answered. They are clearly doing quite a bit of research in making this decision. He was encouraged to continue until he feels comfortable with his decision. He asked me whether I thought he could do that safely without risk of cancer spreading. I told it was likely this had been present for quite a long time and that a couple of weeks to make a decision is safe and appropriate. I asked him to get back to me when he makes a final decision, whether it includes radiotherapy or not. He was given the name of a book, Prostate Cancer, a Nonsurgical Perspective, by Kurt Wallner, MD.

RCW/112 8366
D:11/23/99 12:06 PM
T:11/26/99 2:19:54 PM

ROBERT C. WOLLMAN, MD

Figure 5

PROSTATE CANCER COMPARITIVE MODALITIES
Source: Wessels, Arnold and Henderson Industry Data

	Radical Prostatectomy	External Beam Radiation Tx	Interstitial Brachytherapy
Average Time	3 hours	5 minutes daily for 5 to 6 weeks	45 minutes
Anesthesia	General	None	General / Local or Regional
Complications			
Erectile Dysfunction	50-90%	40-60%	5-15%
Incontinence	2-65%	10-25%	0-2%
Other	Catheterization for 1 to 2 weeks	Rectal complications, Radiation Cystitis	Burning Upon Urination, Difficulty Urinating
Hospital Stay	2-5 Days	Outpatient	Outpatient
Recovery Time	28-42 Days	Variable	2-3 Days
Efficacy	77-95%	50%	79-97%
Payor Cost	$20,000 to $30,000	$12,000 to $15,000	$10,000 to $15,000
Professional Fees	$2,000 to $4,000 for Urologist	$750 Radiation Oncologist	$1,100 Urologist $750 Radiation Oncologist

Figure 6

TABLE V

MOH DECISION MAKING PROCESS

Condition	Rating of Importance	Evaluation of Surgery (x rating)	Evaluation of Internal Radiation (x rating)	Evaluation of External Radiation (x rating)	Cryotherapy IMRT (x rating)	Watchful Waiting (x rating)
Track Record	10	10(100)	9(90)	9(90)	4(40)	8(80)
Longevity	10	10(100)	9(90)	9(90)	9(90)	3(30)
Potency	8	5(40)	9(72)	9(72)	6(64)	10(80)
Continence	9	5(45)	8(72)	7(63)	7(49)	10(90)
Invasiveness	6	1(6)	10(60)	8(48)	10(100)	10(60)
		291	384	363	343	340

Figure 7a and 7b, before and after surgery

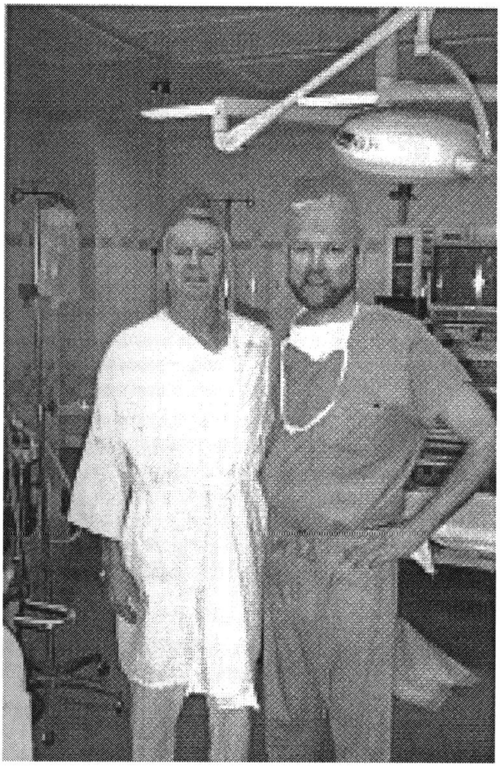

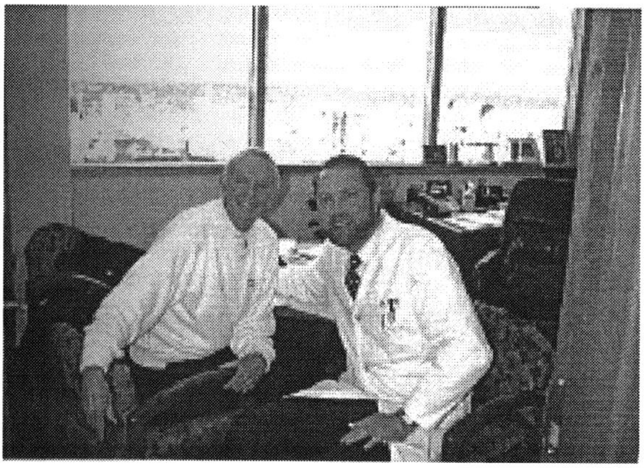

Figure 8

Patients Name:O'Hara, Michael Date: January 27, 2000 [redacted]
Pre Operative Diagnosis: Stage T1c Gleason Score 6 Adenocarcinoma Prostate
Post Operative Diagnosis: Same
Surgeon: Peter Grimm, D.O.
Procedure: Radiosurgical Implantation of I-125 seeds into the Prostate Gland via template guidance

---

Description of procedure: The patient underwent spinal anesthesia and was placed in the dorsal lithotomy position. The perineum was prepped and draped and scrotum secured to the abdominal wall with 3m sterile adhesive drape.

While the patient was undergoing anesthesia, I supervised the loading of the carrier needles with the radioactive seeds. The needles were loaded in the following fashion :

4 needles with 2 seeds per needle 6 needles with 3 seeds per needle
3 needles with 4 seeds per needle 8 needles with 5 seeds per needle
10 needles with 6 seeds per needle 0 needles with 7 seeds per needle

Needles loaded with Rapid Strand and free seeds.
Following this the ultrasound probe was placed into the rectum and the prostate visualized. The template grid pattern was superimposed on the prostate identical to that of the preoperative volume study. After confirmation of the position at the base mid gland and apex, the apparatus was secured and the procedure was begun. Individual needles were inserted into the gland beginning anteriorly and working posteriorly. At each level, the position of the template grid pattern was confirmed. In all 31 needles were inserted into the gland. A total 132 seeds 0.297 per seed were initially placed into the gland.
Additional seeds guided with fluoroscopic assistance.
3 seeds in C 2.5 3 seeds in E 2.5
Seeds recovered at cystoscopy:0
Total Seeds in Prostate : 138
Complications: None
Estimated Blood loss: 15cc
Pubic arch interference: none
Angulation technique required: None
Cystoscopic Findings: No urethral or bladder abnormalities
Flouroscopic Findings: Excellent distribution of Seeds throughout the gland. Seed verification film taken.
Catheter removed prior to discharge.
DISCHARGE MEDICATIONS: Flomax 0.4 QHS, Aleve ii po bid, Bactrim DS BID
Computer authenticated by: Peter Grimm, D.O.

Swedish Hospital Medical Center
Seattle, Washington 98104

OPERATIVE/PROCEDURE REPORT

Figure 9

SEATTLE PROSTATE INSTITUTE

To Our Patients

About a year ago, you elected seed implantation as the treatment for your prostate cancer. One of us participated in your care at Swedish Medical Center in Seattle where you underwent the procedure. We are writing now to ask for your help in carrying out important research on urinary retention. Urinary retention is the inability of urine to pass from the bladder that is caused when the prostate swells, constricting the urethra to the point where the insertion of a catheter is required to drain the bladder until the swelling subsides.

As you surely know, concerns about side effects and complications are extremely important considerations in the minds of men faced with a diagnosis of prostate cancer. The goal of this research is to develop a better understanding of why some men end up needing catheters while others do not. This will enable us to devise ways to minimize the occurrence of urinary retention and, equally as important, to give men a clearer picture of what they can expect during the recovery period following an implant.

The questionnaire on the reverse side of this page should take only a minute or two to complete. For your convenience, we have provided a stamped, return envelope. We recognize that some time has passed since your treatment and that certain details might not be fresh in your mind. Just give the best answer you can. Our statisticians tell us that if enough men take part in this survey, the trends will become clear enough to report on with confidence.

Finally, please be assured that the information you provide will be treated with the utmost confidence. We strictly adhere to state and federal research protocols regarding patient participation and confidentiality. No one will be identified by name during the data analysis or in any subsequent publications and, once processed, all forms will be destroyed. We hope that you will feel secure with these protections and will agree to participate by completing the questionnaire.

On behalf of the entire staff here at SPI, we want to thank you for allowing us to serve you in the past and also to express our sincere wish that you are well and enjoying life

Sincerely,

John Blasko, M.D.   Peter Grimm, D.O.   John Sylvester, M.D.

Figure 10

UroCor, Inc.
840 Research Parkway, Oklahoma City, OK 73104-3699
VOICE (800) 534-9330 FAX (405) 290-4046

Endocrinology Report

FINAL

01-058807S

Report Date: 05/03/01
Specimen: SERUM
Medical Director: Gerard J. O'Dowd, M.D.
Collection Date: 05/02/01 Received Date: 05/03/01 Bar Code: 2314552

Account Information

STANLEY BROSMAN, M.D.
PACIFIC UROLOGY INSTITUTE
KAPLAN, BROSMAN & DECONCINI
2021 SANTA MONICA BLVD, STE 525
SANTA MONICA, CA 90404

Patient Information

Patient Name: OHARA, MIKE
Social Sec. No. [redacted] Phone # [redacted]
Date of Birth: 09/15/1932 Age: 68

Tests Ordered PSA

Test Description	Legend	Test Result	Reference Range	Age-Spec. Ref. Range
Prostate Specific Antigen (EIA) - Total	◆	0.86 ng/ml	0 to 4.0 ng/ml	0 to 4.5 ng/ml

Patient Trend Report

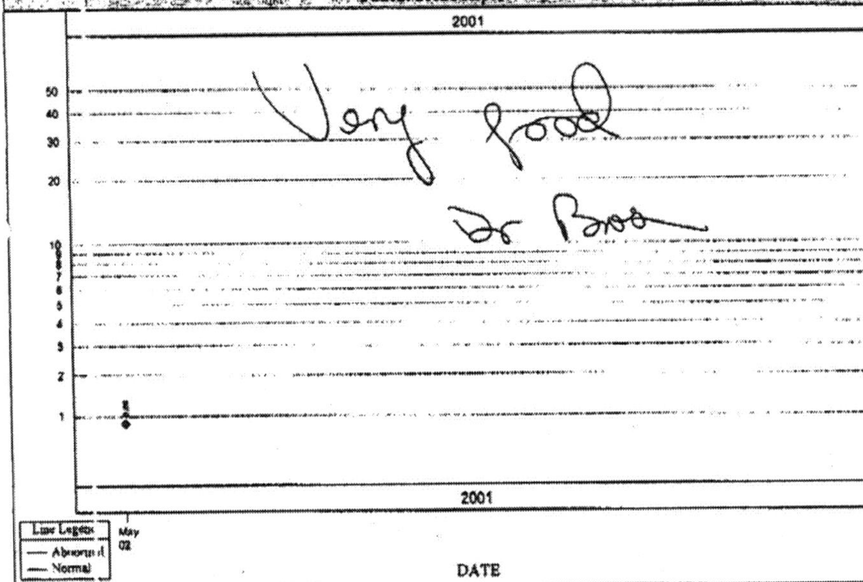

CLIA License Number: 37D0470998 New York License Number: 3970 837021A0

Figure 11

Recent PSA Test Results for Michael O'Hara performed by Dr. Stanley Brosman

5/9/01	.86
9/19/01	1.10
12/11/01	2.10
12/11/01	1.10
7/27/02	.71
10/24/02	.157
8/20/03	.195
2/3/04	.061

Chapter 4

THE ROLE PLAYED BY HMO's CONCERNING PROSTATE CANCER TREATMENT

by Michael O'Hara

Before my failed biopsy, I belonged to one of the nation's largest HMO's. To avoid litigation, I will let both the HMO and their physicians remain anonymous. For five years I enjoyed the services of two bright young internists, even though the process of arranging appointments, waiting to see the physicians and receiving follow up reports seemed to take forever.

When I was informed that my PSA had jumped from 3.6 in June 1988 to 8.89 in September 1999 with a re-test on October 5th yielding 6.65, I was then referred to a HMO urologist for treatment. He reviewed my PSA acceleration and informed me that, in his opinion, a biopsy probably was not necessary because the chances of my having prostate cancer were small. When I asked him what he considered "small" he stated 5% and at the outside 10% (Note: This turned out to be Strike One).

I then contacted my HMO internist and told her of my concern over the urologists recommendation. After a short telephone discussion we mutually agreed, for my personal peace of mind, that I should request a biopsy.

On November 10, 1999, the HMO urologist extracted eighteen strips from my prostate to be tested for cancer cells. The biopsy took approximately forty minutes after which I left the urologist's office nervous and smarting from the procedure and immediately located a rest room on the same floor. My urine was bright red. I became even more concerned when, very upset, I tried to defecate. Once again - a major expulsion of blood occurred! I rushed back through the waiting room and into the urologist's office to report my surprising disaster. His retort was a casual "yes, you're going to bleed like a stuck pig for the next few days." I cannot understand why he did not prepare me for this shock. My urologist continued to treat me with the same disdainful detachment of our first meeting (Strike Two).

Approximately a week later my urologist called me to request a meeting about "a bad news report." He informed me that my prostate biopsy slides had recorded prostate cancer on both sides resulting in a Gleason Score of 3+3 = 6. He indicated that this was the most frequently recorded type score since the PSA test started giving an early warning to prostate cancer patients back in 1988. He further indicated that I would probably be eligible for treatment by most or all of the various prostate cancer procedures.

My urologist then indicated that he was also a surgeon and could take care of my prostate cancer, just as he had for many hundreds of other patients. When I indicated that my brief research had revealed some very serious lifestyle issues concerning loss of potency, and incontinence, I elaborated on my desire to maintain my current lifestyle, playing national caliber Masters Tennis, indoor and Beach Volleyball and Wallyball tournaments. After approximately fifteen minutes of this type of dialogue, his comment was "well then, I guess you shouldn't have surgery after all, because it will make you an old man overnight." The fact that he would pitch me on surgery at first and then turn around and make a statement like that struck me as astonishing. He then gave me a brochure to read called "The Management of Localized Prostate Cancer: A Patient's Guide." It had been prepared by the American Urological Association with an obsolete copyright of 1995! My opinion of this urologist/surgeon had been sinking as a result of the first two strikes and this, as far as I was concerned, was Strike Three and out!

I concluded that, HMO's are fine for economical, general health maintenance, but when you have a serious problem their approach may fall short. This was verified to me in the next recommendation from the HMO urologist. First, he began to sell me on the merits of "watchful waiting." His premise was that the vast majority of Europeans and Asians think that Americans over react. Further research indicated to me that international physicians tend not to recommend the PSA test nor any treatment alternative to this watchful waiting posture and patients consequently follow their physicians' recommendations receiving special diet and herbal remedies instead.

When I probed the longevity issue, i.e. you don't die of prostate cancer unless and only if it escapes the prostate shell, my urologist's comment was that the statistics of the various patients and their treatments vary so much, it is hard to measure which of all the various approaches is best. When I requested a session with the HMO's best physicians specializing in the other treatments, I was told that they supplied external radiation but that Cryotherapy and Brachytherapy were not yet proven enough treatments to be provided.

Before my next HMO appointment, I had met with several of the finest external radiation physicians in the world - Dr. Chris Rose, St. Joseph's Hospital and Dr. Robert Wollman, St. John's Hospital. Both physicians utilize the state-of-the-art treatment called 3D Conformal.

My meeting with the HMO's external radiation specialist started poorly. He proceeded to explain how many thousands of procedures he had personally accomplished. When I asked him if he utilized the equipment that provided the 3D Conformal approach (using three beams instead of two which enables a far more precise delivery system) his answer was "No, we don't have the equipment to provide that system, but we can achieve the same result." Since forty-two radiation treatments would be necessary, I asked him how long each would take using his equipment rather than the more advanced radiation equipment. His answer was "approximately one hour per treatment." I commented that the 3D Conformal treatment time was one to two minutes and indicated that I had been informed by experts that the fatigue factor on the part of the patient and the physician was very important. Then I asked him how a procedure that would call for a total of eighty-four minutes could be compared to one that called for forty-two hours. His reply was an exasperated "Well, it's just as hard on me as it would be on you!"

This reconfirmed my resolution to depart my HMO and never look back. Luckily, being over sixty-five afforded me the opportunity to return my medical rights to Medicare, the "gold standard" of medical support, which has paid for the vast majority of all of my medical expenses concerning prostate cancer, and all other medical treatments I have had since January 1, 2000.

SECTION II

EXPERTS ANALYZE THE LATEST FACTS ABOUT PROSTATE CANCER PREVENTION AND TREATMENT CHOICES

Chapter 5

PROSTATE CANCER PREVENTION INSIGHTS

Dr. Charles "Snuffy" Myers, Jr.

Today's media inundates us with misinformation about health issues of all kinds, especially prostate cancer. In a world of fad diets, thirty-day prostate cancer cures, and miraculous exercise techniques, only the facts based on randomized controlled trials can determine the whole story with any real certainty. However, new information suggests that like prostate cancer, your body's dietary needs are as unique as your fingerprint.

Over the years, I've spent considerable time trying to provide the most accurate information possible on the links between nutrition and prostate cancer in my newsletter, Prostate Forum. As our knowledge of this topic expanded, so did the growing evidence that the same dietary changes that slow prostate cancer growth can also treat heart disease and obesity. This realization led me to the comprehensive cancer care approach implemented in my clinic; I believe that by treating the whole patient, not just his cancer, we can buy a man years of life. The focus on overall health is essential.

We know now that some prostate cancers can be treated by combining a prostate-healthy diet with a regular program of exercise and relaxation. This "Diet & Lifestyle" approach could spare you the often-devastating side effects of treatment while preventing cardiovascular disease. On the flip side, we also know that obesity not only increases your risk of getting a variety of cancers, but also of dying of the disease

I've spent a lot of time discussing diet—in my newsletter; with my patients; and at conferences. Still, I'm struck by the fact that only a small number of the men who come to my Virginia clinic are lean. For many, obesity, and its associated diseases—hypertension, hyperlipidemia, and cardiovascular disease—are much greater threats to their health than prostate cancer will ever be.

There's been an explosion in science's understanding of obesity and of its link to inflammation, cancer, heart disease, and hypertension. This same research has uncovered major links between obesity and prostate cancer that you need to know about.

OBESITY & CANCER

According to the Center for Disease Control, 20% percent of Americans are obese. (Mississippi has by far the heaviest population—25.9%) These statistics are disturbing because despite widespread public health campaigns warning of various weight-related health problems, Americans are quite simply getting fatter and fatter.

We've known for years that obesity leads to a variety of cardiovascular diseases such as heart disease, diabetes, and hypertension. And we've also known that prostate and breast cancers are strongly associated with a high fat diet. But what about other kinds of cancers?

In a recent study published in the New England Journal of Medicine, research suggests that obesity not only increases your risk of getting a variety of cancers, but also of dying of the disease. In this sixteen-year study, researchers examined the relation between body-mass index (BMI) and the risk of death from all cancers and from individual types of cancer.

Obesity is categorized simply by excess body fat. If you have a BMI of over 30 you are obese. An easy way to tell if you are in a high risk weight class is by your waistline (>35 inches for women and >40 for men).

For the heaviest individuals (those with a BMI of at least 40), death rates from all cancers combined were 52% higher for men and 62% higher for women. For men the relative risk of death was 1.52 and for women 1.62. Cancers most affected were: esophagus, colon and rectum, liver, gallbladder, pancreas, kidney, non-Hodgkin's lymphoma, and multiple myeloma. For men, death-rate risk of stomach and prostate cancer increased and for women, breast, uterus, cervix, and ovarian cancer risk increased.

This certainly doesn't bode well for a country in which almost 40% of the citizens are considered either overweight or obese. In fact, the researchers themselves note "the current patterns of overeating in the United States could account for 14% of all deaths from cancer in men and 20% of those in women."

A separate study, by Roberts, Walsh, and Platz, found that obese men had 2.5 times the risk of having prostate cancer than non-obese men. They also discovered that men with advanced disease had a higher BMI than those with localized disease—although when they accounted for age, the difference was not significant.

There's also a relation between BMI and the kind of prostate cancer. Researchers sent a survey that assessed family history to almost 500 men under the age of fifty-five who'd had a radical prostatectomy. Not surprisingly, after controlling for smoking and ethnicity, they found that men who had a family history of prostate cancer were younger at surgery than those who didn't. Interestingly, they also found that these men had a lower risk of a high-grade disease. On the other hand, they found that the risk of a high-grade disease increased as BMI increased, especially in men under age fifty.

So what does this mean? If you reduce your caloric intake, you can significantly reduce your risk of getting and dying from many different kinds of cancer. In fact, recent research suggests that reducing one's calories to 1800 a day can greatly reduce the risk of all health problems later in life.

LOSING THE WEIGHT

Considering the previously mentioned studies, we should all be on a diet. But diet is a very personal endeavor and some people are willing to sacrifice more things than others in the effort to stay healthy. We have advocated a low-fat vegan diet as optimal, but realize this isn't always realistic. Each person has to create a diet that's right—and feasible—for them. As you will see later in this chapter, eating "good" fats promotes health.

Also keep in mind that just because a meal is vegan doesn't mean it's lower in fat or in calories than traditional options. Food like peanut butter, nuts, and some kinds of bean curd are very high in calories, which can be confusing if you're trying to lose weight. Even olive oil is high in calories. We encourage you to become diligent label readers and to carefully record your fat and calorie intake.

This point brings us to the controversial issue of carbohydrates. As most of you know, the Atkins diet has been making headlines since the seventies. The Atkins diet eliminates starch in favor of high protein, high-fat foods. Now, it may be true that you'll lose weight on this diet. In fact, a new study confirms that reducing carbohydrates can help you lose weight. So it's a good idea to reduce the amount of foods like bread, pasta, and potatoes that you eat. But increasing your intake of animal fats will only lead to more health problems, such as prostate cancer, down the line. If you want to lose weight choose a low carbohydrate, low-cal, healthy protein diet. Healthy proteins include egg whites, fish, skinless chicken breast, and beans. Pork chops, on the other hand, are a decidedly unhealthy protein. Remember: pork is not the other white meat but is as dangerous as beef.

There are those who argue that life simply isn't worth living if you're reduced to a diet low in animal fat. But such a diet doesn't have to taste bad—as evidenced by the plethora of cookbooks and cooking shows available today. And considering the numerous health problems involved with a high animal fat diet, ignoring the warning of countless health professionals could mean shortening your life span or facing severe debilitation. Now, I've always aimed to give you accurate health information that will help you live longer and happier lives. What good does it do you to survive prostate cancer only to have your leg amputated six months later because of severe obesity-related diabetes?

THE OBESITY CRISIS

Americans today confront an obesity pandemic unprecedented in human history. In the late 1960s, adult-onset diabetes was commonly found in people over 50 who'd gradually gained weight during their adult years. Now we're seeing a rapid increase in the incidence of adult-onset diabetes among those in their 20s, and, more recently, among high school students! This increase in diabetes among the young is directly linked to a rapid increase in obesity between the onset of puberty and age 30. The consequences of this epidemic are far-reaching and the causes significantly ingrained within our fast-food, quick-fix culture.

Here's the bad news: there's no easy way to stay thin. In fact, most of us find it very difficult to lose weight and maintain a healthy BMI. This is why there are so many diet books on the market, each one claiming to have finally solved the problem. We also have the absurd situation that there is absolutely no agreement among "experts" about the best way to lose weight. Dr. Atkins was convinced that carbohydrates were the major problem and the solution was a diet high in fat and protein and low in carbohydrate. Dr. Ornish is convinced that a diet needs to be very low in fat, moderate in protein content, and high in complex carbohydrates. Among those in the bodybuilding world, it's standard to advocate a diet very high in protein, adequate in carbohydrate, and low in fat. Each of these approaches has attracted celebrities and fans who feel that only one of these approaches work for them. But the good news is that scientific evidence shows that humans differ markedly in how they respond to fat and carbohydrate.

Some may lose weight best with carbohydrate restriction while others seem to benefit most from a high carbohydrate low fat diet. There's simply no way that a diet like Atkins, South Beach, or The Zone will ever work for all Americans: <u>the path to weight loss is as individual as DNA.</u>

Media and scientific scrutiny on the subject of diet and weight loss has sparked a flurry of new studies that are rapidly revolutionizing our understanding of obesity and its consequences. Investigators have discovered a range of new hormones that interact to maintain body weight. Hormones such as IGF-1, leptin, ghrelin, resistin, and adiponectin have all been found to play important roles in controlling body fat accumulation. Two of these, leptin and IGF-1, are known to play a role in prostate cancer progression and leptin has also been shown to be one of the factors that link obesity with wide spread inflammation of the blood vessels and other tissues.

CALORIE RESTRICTION & PROSTATE CANCER

Scientific research has identified a range of new hormones that regulate eating and getting fat. One of the best studied of these is leptin. The discovery of leptin started when scientists developed of a strain of mice with a genetic predisposition to obesity. These mice don't produce the protein we now call leptin. When these mice are injected with leptin they lose a significant amount of body fat, confirming that it was the original lack of leptin that led to obesity. Later, researchers showed that leptin is produced by fat cells in increasing quantities as they fill with lipid. The result is that gaining body fat increases production of a hormone that further limits fat production by decreasing feeding and other metabolic changes. In contrast, fasting caused a rapid decrease in leptin production in mice.

For a while, it looked as if leptin injections would be an effective way to treat obesity, but this hope waned as it became obvious that leptin did much more than reduce body fat. Obesity is associated with increased inflammation of the arteries and other tissues. And the most convenient measure of this inflammation is the ultrasensitive C-reactive protein test (CRP). An elevated CRP result has now been shown to be as important as the serum total cholesterol count in predicting who is at risk for heart disease. And we now know that leptin stimulates inflammation by releasing a protein called tumor necrosis factor (TNF) and a protein called IL-6. (It is now thought that many of the adverse consequences of obesity are the consequences of chronic elevation of leptin.)

Both leptin and IL-6 stimulate the growth of human prostate cancer and elevated blood levels of either protein are associated with a poor prostate cancer prognosis. In particular, leptin stimulates the growth of hormone-resistant prostate cancer. Thus, leptin is directly or indirectly linked with obesity, inflammation, cardiovascular disease, and prostate cancer progression.

In humans, calorie restriction leads to a rapid drop in blood leptin levels as well as levels of TNF, IL6, and CRP. We had previously mentioned that the most successful programs for weight loss all incorporate diet and exercise. Research has repeatedly shown that exercise reduces circulating leptin, TNF, IL6, and CRP. The longer you exercise, the greater the reduction of blood leptin levels. In fact, exercising for more than one hour appears to be necessary for maximal reduction. Ultramarathoners, runners who compete in races up to 50 or 100 miles, carry this process to the ultimate and very dramatic suppression of leptin.

INSULIN-LIKE GROWTH FACTOR 1 (IGF1)

In the laboratory, IGF1 stimulates the growth and survival of prostate cancer cells. And men with elevated IGF1 levels are at an increased risk for the development of prostate cancer. In hormone-resistant prostate cancer, one of the most common genetic changes involves those that would increase the effectiveness of IGF1 in promoting the growth and survival of the cancer cells. A number of treatment approaches target IGF1 and its effects on prostate cancer cells. Sandostatin is a drug that suppresses IGF1 production and has been reported to reverse hormone-resistance. The anti-inflammatory drug Celebrex has been reported to block akt, a protein that plays a significant role in the changes IGF1 causes in cancer cells. Celebrex has been reported to kill human prostate cancer cells in the laboratory. Rapamycin blocks a protein called mTOR, another protein used by IGF1 to promote prostate cancer cell survival. This drug has also been reported to reverse hormone-resistance.

But there are much simpler ways to reduce IGF1 level□□s. Elevated IGF1, as well as the proteins we've just discussed that appear to be involved in prostate cancer progression, are also involved in aging and you can alter them with diet. Calorie restriction can reduce IGF1 levs and its effects—which is a critical step in promoting a longer lifespan. In fact, calorie restriction's ability to block IGF1 and its actions is thought to be one of the major mechanisms by which it slows aging.

One of the disadvantages of an Atkins-like, high protein diet (particularly one rich in animal protein) is that it stimulates IGF1 production. If you switch from a diet rich in animal protein to a moderate protein diet from plant sources you can significantly decrease your IGF1 levels. The Okinawans and Kalenjin diets both can be expected to result in reduced IGF1 levels compared to that of the typical American. Our book, Eating Your Way To Better Health describes a diet likely to decrease IGF1 levels, especially if coupled with calorie restriction.

PROSTATE-HEALTHY FATS

Not too long ago we were all told that the best diet was high in carbohydrates and low in fats. More recently, physicians are recommending that we emphasize low-glycemic carbohydrates because they raise blood sugar the least. This low-glycemic diet pattern is the basis for a range of popular diets, including those promoted by Drs. Pritikin, Ornish, and MacDougal, as well as the Macrobiotic enthusiasts.

More recently, those involved in nutrition research, as well as those who use diet to manage diabetes, heart disease, hypertension, obesity, and cancer, have questioned this high-carb and low-fat recommendation. Several observations have led to reservations about low-fat dieting. First, humans evolved as hunter-gatherers and most hunter-gatherers consume a diet rich in animal products when they are available. Many argue that humans have adapted to a diet rich in animal proteins and fats through the course of evolution.

I'm not particularly impressed with this line of reasoning because for most of human history, the average life span was less than 40. Today we're concerned with finding a diet that yields optimal health for those over 50. This is not something that evolution would have addressed because it only selects for those things that affect human reproduction. In other words, we are now trying to ensure humans attain a life span beyond that seen in hunter-gatherer societies.

I'm much more impressed with the growing list of useful clinical trials that demonstrate the health benefits of the Mediterranean diet, in which fat typically comprises between 30-40% of calories. One excellent example of this evidence is the Lyon Diet Heart Study. This clinical trial compared a modified version of the diet consumed on the island of Crete with the level 1 diet recommended by the American Heart Association. The level 1 diet places modest limits on dietary fat and cholesterol intake, but is based on the eating habits of the typical American or Northern European. The Mediterranean diet limited meat consumption to fish and poultry and emphasized fruits, vegetables, and grains. Participants were encouraged to use olive oil as their primary fat source. They were also encouraged to drink red wine in moderation. There were 605 participants with coronary heart disease who were randomized to these two diets. After four years, subjects on the Mediterranean diet had a 56% reduction in total deaths, 61% reduction in cancers of all types, as well as a close to 50% reduction in heart attacks. While these results are impressive, it is even more important that the benefits shown in this study have been repeatedly confirmed.

You may well ask: How can the Mediterranean diet be healthy despite its high fat content? The answer is actually simple: there are fats that are actually good for you and the Mediterranean diet happens to emphasize just those fats. In contrast, the diet common in America and Northern Europe emphasizes fats that have an adverse impact on health, increasing the risk of obesity, heart disease, hypertension, and cancer.

ADDING HEALTHY FATS TO YOUR DIET

Switching from dangerous to healthy fats can be a daunting task for those of us raised on a traditional American or European diet. Luckily, there are a variety of texts that can help you create healthy and tasty meals.

Eating Your Way to Better Health
by Rose Sgarlat Myers, Charles Myers & Sara Sgarlat Steck

Our staple nutrition guide will help you modify the Mediterranean diet for its maximum benefit for prostate cancer patients. The cooking style focuses on dishes that are simple to prepare. Many of the recipes come from my wife's Sicilian family.

Mediterranean Grains and Greens:
A Book of Savory, Sun-Drenched Recipes
by Paula Wolfert

Paula Wolfert is one of the best cookbook authors around and specializes in Mediterranean cooking. Actually, any Mediterranean cookbook by Paula Wolfert is worth reading, but this book is very special because it introduces Americans to the healthful, Mediterranean custom of blending whole grains and greens.

The Mediterranean Diet Cookbook
by Nancy Harmon Jenkins

This is a comprehensive presentation of Mediterranean cooking.

The Italian Country Table
by Lynne Rossetto Kasper

This is a wonderful introduction to simple country food you'd encounter in the farms and small towns of Italy. It also contains fascinating discussions of regional customs and how they manifest in cooking styles.

Cooking by Hand
by Paul Bertolli

Paul Bertolli is Executive Chef at Oliveto Restaurant in Oakland, California, where my youngest daughter worked as a line cook for several years. This is one of the best Italian restaurants in America and was rated as such in a recent issue of the Wall Street Journal. Bertolli's cookbook is very unusual because it is composed of essays on various elements of the Mediterranean diet, especially focusing on enhancing the best possible ingredients. The end result yields recipes that are both elegant and simple. He even includes a discussion about how to cure fresh olives.

Olives & Olive Oil

Olives play a central role in Mediterranean cuisine and are responsible for the high fat content of the diet. As a result, research on the health benefits of the Mediterranean diet has naturally focused on olives and olive oil.

There are a number of reasons why the olive is so important in Mediterranean cuisine. For one thing, olive trees grow well in soil that is otherwise too dry and too rocky for most other plants. The success of early farming as it developed in the eastern Mediterranean was based on its ability to provide calories in a form that was easily stored so it could sustain human life between harvests. Thus, grains and legumes such as wheat, barley, lentils, and chickpeas played an important role in these early farming communities. The olive complemented these grains and legumes by providing a practical way to store fat calories between harvests.

Olives are also intensely bitter because of their high polyphenolic antioxidant concentration. Olives can be rendered palatable, though, by extracting these embittering compounds in salty water or through other curing methods. It's also true that salt blocks the human tongue's ability to taste the bitter compounds that remain. The combination of high salt content and abundant polyphenolic antioxidants acts to preserve the olive.

The olive is unusual in that it yields high-quality oil when crushed and pressed under primitive conditions. Most other oils available today are extracted using high temperatures or organic solvents such as hexane—methods unavailable to early humans. Keep in mind that all oils are susceptible to oxidation: they can turn rancid for example. Olive oil, however, is less susceptible because it's protected by its high concentration of antioxidants like vitamin E and polyphenols. This is why olive oil can be stored successfully for long periods of time—as long as it's protected from light and heat. Of course, the fact that it could easily be stored for so long only furthered its importance in early farming societies. The fact that the taste of olive oil itself melds so well with many of the grains and vegetables that make up Mediterranean cuisine make it an ideal lipid for the healthy dieter.

There are a number of other factors that make olive oil better for your health than most oils currently available in America. One of the most important factors is that the predominant fatty acid in olive oil is monounsaturated oleic acid. Diets rich in monounsaturated oleic acid are associated with a reduced risk of breast and prostate cancer. There is even evidence that this fatty acid reduces arterial inflammation and damage.

The polyphenolic antioxidants that make fresh olives bitter appear to play an important role in reducing oxidative damage to your body. These polyphenolic antioxidants are found in the greatest concentration in brined, or salt-cured, olives. Polyphenolic antioxidants are also present in olive oil; they give extra virgin olive oil its characteristic taste. In contrast, antioxidant concentration is very low in the "lite" olive oils available to American consumers. As you will see, these "lite" oils have their uses, even though they are low in antioxidants.

Phytosterols are another class of chemicals found in olives and olive oil that have a potential health benefit. Phytosterols are plant chemicals similar to cholesterol in structure but cannot be converted into cholesterol and don't cause arterial deposits. The predominant phytosterol in olives is beta-sitosterol. Researchers have extensively studied beta-sitosterol and have shown that it blocks the gut's ability to absorb cholesterol. Beta-sitosterol effectively lowers cholesterol in patients with mild hypercholesterolemia. In fact, a recent randomized controlled trial showed that the combination of beta-sitosterol, Metamucil, soy protein, and almonds was as effective as the cholesterol-lowering drug Zocor in the treatment of hypercholesterolemia. Beta-sitosterol also appears to have a favorable impact on the prostate gland and has been successfully used to treat benign prostatic hyperplasia (BPH).

But there are some practical issues you need to know about as you incorporate olive oil into your diet. While the phytosterol and antioxidant content is greatest in unfiltered extra virgin olive oil, this form also has the most intense olive flavor, which some people find objectionable. Even some olive oil lovers find the flavor too strong for baked goods. Also, extra virgin olive oil breaks down at a fairly low temperature, making it a poor choice for sautéing or frying food at high heat. The newly available "lite" olive oils not only have a much more neutral taste, but also tolerate much higher temperatures without breaking down or smoking. These oils still have monounsaturated oleic acid and provide some of the benefits of extra virgin olive oil, even though, as we discussed earlier, the antioxidant concentration is lower than extra virgin oils.

And olive oil makes an excellent carrier for other important nutrients. Lycopene, the red pigment in tomatoes, is absorbed much better if olive oil is added to the cooked tomatoes. This is true for other carotenoids such as lutein, a carotenoid known to protect vision and lessen the risk of prostate cancer.

There are also health benefits associated with eating allium vegetables like onions and garlic. In Mediterranean cooking, garlic and onions are commonly crushed or chopped and then immersed in olive oil. The aromatic chemicals in garlic and onions are released after injury, but can escape into the air. By mixing garlic or onions with olive oil, these health-giving chemicals are trapped by the olive oil. It is important to note, however, that the health benefits associated with allium vegetables are most potent when consumed with minimal cooking.

Researchers have clearly established, through large-scale randomized controlled trials, the safety and efficacy of olive oil consumption. The biological basis for the health-promoting aspects of this oil rests on its rich oleic acid content, as well as its high concentration of beta-sitosterol and polyphenolic antioxidants. You don't need to be a chemist, however, to know a good healthy meal when you see one.

Almonds & Almond Oil

Almonds are an important component of Mediterranean cuisine. In fact, before tomatoes arrived from the New World, Italian pasta sauces were commonly modeled after traditional pesto and consisted of various nuts, olive oil, and pureed greens. In many of these dishes, almonds played a major role.

It's now clear that almonds and other nuts play a key role in the healthy properties of the Mediterranean diet, as a recent study by Sabate, et al. demonstrated. Patients on a basic heart-healthy diet were divided into three groups, which were fed diets in which almonds contributed 0, 10, and 20% of the daily calories. As the almond content of the diet increased, total cholesterol and LDL-cholesterol (or "bad" cholesterol) decreased. Since HDL-cholesterol ("good" cholesterol) did not decrease, the ratio of LDL to HDL cholesterol shifted in a healthy direction.

In a second study by Wien, et al., overweight and obese adults were placed on one of two diets. One was a calorie-restricted diet in which close to 50% of calories were derived from complex carbohydrates. In the other group, 84 grams of almonds replaced an equivalent number of calories from complex carbohydrates. While both groups consumed the same number of calories a day, the patients who ate almonds lost more weight and had a greater decline in waist size and blood pressure. Insulin resistance (the underlying abnormality that causes obesity and diabetes) decreased by 66% in the patients eating almonds compared to 35% in those eating complex carbohydrates alone. Among patients with adult-onset diabetes, 96% of those eating almonds reduced the amount of diabetes medication they needed, while only 50% of people eating complex carbohydrates reduced their medication.

This is just a limited sample of the growing literature demonstrating important health benefits associated with almond consumption. But why are almonds so good for your health? As with olive oil, almonds are rich in monounsaturated oleic acid. In fact, almonds have essentially the same level of oleic acid as olive oil. Almonds are also a rich source of phytosterols, especially beta-sitosterol, which plays an important role in effecting favorable blood cholesterol levels. Finally, almonds are a rich source of antioxidants, but it's important to note that much of the antioxidant content is found in the skin of the nut.

The specific antioxidants in almonds differ significantly from those in olives and olive oil and there are reasons to think that almond antioxidants may in fact complement those found in olives. Almonds are a significant source of quercetin and related compounds. Quercetin has anticancer activity and markedly increases cancer cell sensitivity to radiation therapy (re Prostate Forum authority source).

While almonds have not been specifically tested as a treatment for prostate disease, their high content of monounsaturated fat and phytosterols (especially quercetin) make it likely that <u>they will have a beneficial impact on BPH and PCa.</u>

But if you decide to incorporate almonds into your diet, there are several issues you need to consider. It's best if you eat almonds with their skins on because of the skin's nutritional properties. You also need to make sure the skin is intact; there's a fungus that can infect damaged nuts, which produces a cancer-causing chemical called aflatoxin. While this is a particularly severe problem with peanuts, almonds damaged by insects also produce aflatoxin. I think it's better to use raw rather than roasted almonds; the roasting process damages the antioxidant content and can cause oxidation of the unsaturated fats in the nut.

Almond oil is also available and has many of the health benefits associated with olive oils. But almond oil has a very mild flavor, making it more attractive than olive oil in situations in which the strong flavor of olives presents a problem. I've found almond oil makes excellent vinaigrettes when combined with champagne or sherry vinegar. I think it's superior to olive oil for fruit-based vinaigrettes, such as raspberry or cherry.

Almonds are commonly ground into a butter that can be an excellent replacement for peanut butter. I find it has a richer, nuttier flavor that goes well with toast. It makes an excellent nut and jelly sandwich. Our local Whole Foods store has a machine that custom grinds almonds into butter so you can be assured it's fresh and not adulterated. You may find this in a store near you. Because it's rich in unsaturated fat, almond butter can spoil quickly if not cared for properly. I only buy what I am likely to eat over the next week or so and make sure to store it in the refrigerator.

Avocados & Avocado Oil

Avocados are a rich source of oleic acid (75%) and, like olives and almonds, can reduce total cholesterol and LDL-cholesterol. Unlike olives and almonds, however, avocados can increase HDL-cholesterol and reduce triglycerides. Avocados appear to be most effective in cholesterol control if they're combined with a reduction in overall calorie consumption. They're beneficial when added to a diet rich in complex carbohydrates and when the calories added by avocados are matched by a decrease in carbohydrate calories.

Avocado contains the phytosterol beta-sitosterol. In fact, it's one of the richest sources of beta-sitosterol—433 mg per 100 grams of avocado oil. This may well explain why it has a greater impact on blood cholesterol than either olive or almond oil. Again, since beta-sitosterol appears to have a favorable impact on prostate disease, avocados and avocado oil may well be beneficial.

Avocados not only contain the same antioxidants as olives and almonds, but they also contain agents called persenones that are very active in suppressing inflammation. As a result, avocados can decrease the severity of a sunburn and appear to be very active at protecting the liver.

Avocado oil has recently become available and appears to have the same health benefits as olive oil. Because it has both a high concentration of oleic acid and low levels of polyunsaturated fats, avocado oil is very stable at high temperatures. In fact, it takes more than 500°F for the oil to break down, making it suitable for frying or sautéing. The oil is an attractive golden yellow color and its flavor is both nutty and buttery, which makes for an excellent salad dressing.

Hazelnuts & Hazelnut Oil

Hazelnuts (or filberts) contain 70-80% oleic acid and are also low in both saturated and polyunsaturated fats. As with other foods rich in oleic acid, these nuts decrease total and LDL-cholesterol.

While hazelnuts contain antioxidants and beta-sitosterol, the levels of both are less than those found in olives, almonds, or avocados.

Hazelnut oil is widely available and truly delightful. It has a nice nutty flavor reminiscent of sesame seed oil, which I don't recommend because of its high concentration of the polyunsaturated linoleic acid. I've found that hazelnut oil is a nice substitute for sesame seed paste in hummus recipes.

As with other nuts, hazelnuts are susceptible to fungal toxins such as aflatoxin. You can reduce the risk of consuming this toxin by only purchasing nuts with intact skins that show no insect damage. It's also important that farmers promptly dry the nuts after harvest. Turkey, where humid, rainy weather during the harvest season can create problems, produces approximately 70% of the hazelnuts in the world. California hazelnuts, on the other hand, are more consistent in quality and are easy to find.

Macadamia Nuts & Macadamia Oil

Macadamia nuts have the highest concentration of monounsaturated fat of any nut (80%) coupled with low levels of both polyunsaturated and saturated fats. Interestingly, oleic acid comprises only 50% of the fat; palmitoleic acid makes up for the remaining 30% of the monounsaturated fat. Unfortunately, palmitoleic acid doesn't have the same health benefits as oleic acid. Nevertheless, recent clinical trials demonstrated that macadamia nut consumption does decrease total and LDL-cholesterol while increasing HDL-cholesterol.

Macadamia nut oil is also available. As with the other oils high in monounsaturated fat, it's quite stable in the presence of high heat, making it great for sautéing. It has a very neutral flavor, making it suitable for use in settings where the absence of distinct flavor is desired.

Designer Nuts & Oils?

Oils high in monounsaturated fats are healthy for you and much more stable than polyunsaturated fats. Plus, they're as heat stable as saturated fats or those that have been chemically altered by hydrogenation. The latter are now called "trans fats" which have been shown to have a very adverse impact on cardiovascular health. Thus, there is now a great demand for oils high in monounsaturated fats for use in the fast food industry and in the preparation of baked goods because they allow the elimination of both saturated and trans fats. This has resulted in extensive research designed to develop strains of peanuts, soybeans, safflower, cottonseed, and canola that are high in oleic acid and low in polyunsaturated fat. In each case, the resulting products are more stable than the original forms with lower oleic acid. For example, in the case of peanuts, the shelf life of roasted peanuts goes from 2 months for standard varieties to 37 months for those with high oleic acid content. I must stress that none have been tested in properly designed clinical trials. (I personally won't eat any of these designer nuts or oils until they are proven safe.)

THE BOTTOM LINE

Olive oil has been a staple in my diet for years, but, based on the research I've outlined in this issue, I've started to incorporate avocado and hazelnut oils into my culinary practices.

For more information call 800-305-2432 or visit www.prostateforum.com.

Chapter 6

DIET AND PROSTATE CANCER FROM DR. MARK MOYAD

by Michael O'Hara

I tried to motivate Dr. Mark Moyad, one of the world's leading expert on preventative measures concerning Prostate Cancer, to write a chapter for this book. He is a strong advocate of the Prostate Cancer Research Institute (PCRI) and I am also closely affiliated with this leading national dispenser of information on this important subject.

After several months of exchanging information with Dr. Moyad, it became clear that he was far too busy treating patients and giving speeches around the country to prepare what I needed. After considerable bartering, we settled on letting me take some of the pertinent information from his recent book, "The A through Z Guide to Supplements, Alternative Medicines, and Personal Choices" which I would strongly recommend for your follow up reading.

Dr. Moyad starts that portion of his book by requesting that you do not use supplement or alternative medicine therapies as a substitute for medical treatment. You should discuss their use with your doctor and, if acceptable, use in combination with conventional treatment(s). Also, if a specific dose is not included it is because a safe general recommendation has not been determined. Answers to whether or not the medical evidence supports the use of therapies are listed as: YES, NO, or MAYBE.

One of only two subjects that received a YES dealt with EXERCISE, WALKING, AND DEPRESSION TO REDUCE YOUR CHANCES OF DISEASE AND PROSTATE CANCER PROGRESSION OR DEALING WITH RELATED DEPRESSION.

Two large and recent studies have found that walking (six times a month for 30 minutes or more) or a walking-related exercise have been shown to decrease an individual's chances of early death. Another recent study has shown a potentially lower risk of advanced Prostate Cancer among men involved in regular and vigorous activities, i.e. walking, golf, tennis, swimming, etc. Other studies have shown that moderate exercise may reduce testosterone levels in the body and stimulate the immune system, while intense exercise can cause immune suppression. Regular, moderate exercise is very important to good health! Several medical articles have reported that any type of exercise may help reduce depression. In fact, it has been found that exercise may be as effective as psychotherapy in some cases. (Although this does not mean you should substitute your psychotherapy for exercise.)

The second YES dealt with HEALTHY BODY WEIGHT

Increased weight can increase your chances of diabetes(type two), high cholesterol, and heart disease, and has been associated with a number of hormonal-dependent cancers, such as PROSTATE, breast and ovarian cancer. Individuals with abnormal weight of the upper body have also been found to experience unfavorable changes in hormonal levels. For example, the amount of sex hormone-binding globulin can be reduced by added weight, which means free testosterone levels can increase. In addition, there is recent evidence to show that other factors related to weight gain could increase Prostate Cancer growth. Regardless, there is little doubt that maintaining a healthy body weight is also healthy for you overall.

The following have undergone limited research to date. No testing has been done to determine their effect on Prostate Cancer. Further testing needs to be completed prior to their use. Please watch for their test results.

Bilberry - for circulation
Bee pollen and royal jelly for general health
Benecol and Take Control margarine spreads to reduce cholesterol
Cancell (also known as Entelev and Cantron) cancer treatment
Carob (and bananas) to reduce diarrhea
Cat's Claw for an immune boost
Electromagnetic fields from power lines - as cancer causing
Noni juice or supplements from the plant Morinda Caitrifolia from Hawaii - to promote health
Octacosanol for fatigue
Pregnenolone - which can be converted to DHEA, testosterone, and other hormones - may help combat aging problems (stay away from this)
Qi gong as an exercise may be healthy.
Rosemary for cancer protection
Silicon from high-fiber foods - for general health
Thymic protein A - for an immune boost
Wheat grass for general health
Yohimoe for impotence

The next category Dr. Moyad reveals to us is the MAYBE area, which I will describe in less detail (for more detail I will refer you to his book).

MEDITERRANEAN DIET

The Mediterranean is filled with plant-based foods, such as fruits, vegetables, nuts, seeds, breads, potatoes, and cereals. Moderation is recommended for meat consumption, dairy, and alcohol. Fresh fruit is a common dessert; olive oil is a primary source of fat; and garlic, onions, and other items are commonly used in recipes. The Mediterranean diet is also high in omega-3 fatty acids, low in saturated fats, and high in dietary vitamins (not supplements) such as the B-vitamins. Other factors related to this diet that are not commonly mentioned are regular walking and frequent social gatherings. Recent clinical studies (the Lyon Diet Heart Study) have demonstrated that this type of diet is associated with large reductions ion incidence of early deaths, CANCERS, and heart disease. Whether or not this type of diet will reduce the number of clinically significant Prostate Cancers remains to be seen, but it is promising.

MICROBIOTIC DIET

There has been one direct study of the effect of a macrobiotic diet after a diagnosis of advanced Prostate Cancer (stage D2, or bone metastaisi). There were 18 patients in this study, 9 of whom followed the diet for at least three months. The average survival time for the patients in the study was 177 months (more than 14 years), while the average survival time for the control group (the group not participating in the diet) was 91 monrhs (more than 7 years). Although this was only a small trial the results show hope for advanced Prostate Cancer patients. The only drawback is that a macrobiotic diet can be very difficult to follow. Please ask your local bookseller to locate books on macrobiotic diets for you.

CLINICAL TRIALS FOR PROSTATE CANCER

There are a number of clinical trials being conducted around the country for Prostate Cancer patients. For example, at the UCLA Center for Human Nutrition 40 patients with Prostate Cancer who had a radical prostatectomy (with a Gleason score of 7 or greater) and an undetectable PSA after surgery were placed either in a dietary change group or in a control group. The dietary change group maintain a high fiber diet that emphasizes fruit, vegetables, cereals, grains and 40 grams of soy protein isolate daily. No more than 15% of their daily calories come from fat. Results of this study will be published at a point in the future.

Dr. Ornish is conducting a study of men with Prostate Cancer who have a PSA of greater than 4. All were either assigned to the experimental or control groups. The experimental group is on a low-fat diet supplemented with soy and antioxidents, moderate aerobic exercise, stress management, and psychosocial support. In the first year of this trial men in the experimental group experienced declines in their PSA that were larger than those of the control group. In men with initial PSA levels greater than 10, both groups experienced an increase in their PSA levels, although these increases were not as great in the experimental group. Results will be published in the future.

OTHER DIETS

There are many other potentially healthy diets depending on your situation, i.e. Dean Ornish Diet, Pritikin Diet, Zone Diet - although you may wish to reduce fat intake to 20%. You can locate books on these diets at your local bookstore.

Alpha-Linolenic Acid (An Omega-3 Fatty Acid)
For Prostate Cancer prevention and treatment, from flaxseed and canola oil, not from meat.

Black Cohosh
For treating hot flashes due to hormone ablation treatment, not for Prostate Cancer prevention and treatment.

Boron
For bone health from osteoporosis from hormone ablation treatment for Prostate Cancer, not for Prostate Cancer treatment.

Calcium
For the prevention of osteoporosis from hormonal ablation treatment for Prostate Cancer, not for the prevention and treatment of Prostate Cancer.

Cenestin (soy and yam supplement)
For the treatment of hot flashes from Prostate Cancer treatment, but not for the prevention and/or treatment of Prostate Cancer.

Chamomile

For hot flashes and stomach upset from chemotherapy, but not for Prostate Cancer prevention and treatment.

Chasteberry

For hot flashes from hormone ablation treatment for Prostate Cancer, but not for Prostate Cancer prevention and treatment.

Dandelion

As a liver tonic for antiandrogen therapy for Prostate Cancer, but not for Prostate Cancer prevention and treatment.

DMSO (dimethyl sulfoxide) and MSM (methylsulfonylmethane)

For the treatment of some types of pain from Prostate Cancer, but not for the prevention and/or treatment of Prostate Cancer.

Fish Oil Capsules

For gaining weight for some advanced Prostate Cancer patients, but not for Prostate Cancer prevention and treatment.

Fructose

For the prevention and treatment of Prostate Cancer.

Ginger

For the prevention of nausea from chemotherapy for Prostate Cancer, but not for Prostate Cancer prevention and treatment.

Ginseng

To offset fatigue from Prostate Cancer treatment, but not for prevention or treatment.

Goldenseal

In the future for side effects due to antiandrogen treatment for Prostate Cancer, but not for prevention and treatment.

Hydrazine Sulfate

For advanced Prostate Cancer patients with extreme weight loss, but not for prevention or progression.

IGF-1 (Also known as Insulin-like Growth Factor)

In the future as a test to determine your risk of Prostate Cancer.

L-Arginine

For the treatment of some types of Erectile Dysfunction, but not for the prevention and/or treatment of Prostate Cancer.

Licorice

For hot flashes from hormone ablation or side effects from antiandrogen treatment for Prostate Cancer, but not prevention and treatment.

N-Acetylcysteine

For severe loss of muscle mass associated with advanced Prostate Cancer, but not for prevention and treatment.

Oltipraz

For the prevention of Prostate Cancer

Quercetin

For the prevention and/or treatment of Non-Bacterial Chronic Prostates, but not for the prevention and treatment of |Prostate Cancer.

Red Clover

For Prostate Cancer prevention and treatment.

SAM-e (S-Adenosylmethionine)

For the treatment of depression from a Prostate Cancer diagnosis, but not for prevention and treatment.

Silymarin (Milk Thisle)
For patients on prescribed antiandrogens, but not for Prostate Cancer prevention or progression.

Turmeric
For hot flashes from hormonal ablation treatment for Prostate Cancer, but not for prevention and treatment.

Valerian
For stress, anxiety, and insomnia after diagnosis of Prostate Cancer, but not for prevention and treatment

Water (bottled or tap)
No special preference right now for drinking bottled or tap water. Oveere the past few years, sales of bottled water have increased 400%. Today more than one in five homes in the U.S. uses bottled water regularly. The focus should be on five minerals in your water for health reasons.

Fluoride - important for strengthening bones. Fluoride in tap water has been associated with some major decreases in tooth decay and cavities in certain parts of the United States.

Calcium - can lower your risk of osteoporosis.

Magnesium - may be essential to proper cardiovascular function. Higher levels have been associated with a reduced risk of sudden death.

Sodium - should not be consumed in large quantities. It has been associated with high blood pressure, or hypertension.

Potassium - has been associated with a lower risk of stroke.

Since the above illuminated the MAYBES, it is also important to identify the NO'S, since they are not recommended to use in the prevention and treatment of Prostate Cancer. They are:

Alcohol, Aloe Vera, Amino Acid Supplements, Androstenedione, Arachidonic Acid (an Omega-6 Fatty Acid), Astragalus, Beta-Glucana (and mushroom supplements), Bioflavonolds, Caffeine, Coffee, and Chocolate, Conjugated Linoleic Acid (CLA), Dong Qua, Echinacea, Ephedra, Raspberry.

Once again, for additional detailed information on all of the above, please refer to Dr. Mark Moyad's terrific book: THE A THROUGH Z GUIDE TO SUPPLEMENTS, ALTERNATIVE MEDICINES, AND PERSONAL CHOICE.

There have only been a few studies of tap water and cancer risk. For example, in a study from Spain, gastric cancer rates were higher in men and women who had high levels of nitrates in their drinking water. It was also found that Prostate Cancer rates were higher in men whose water contained higher amounts of nitrates. Please remember that there have been only a few studies = no final results have been determined to date.

To have your tap water tested in your house, call the Enviornmental Protection Agency at 800-426-4791. Operators can direct you to a state-certified agency that provides you with a list of local testing laboratories. Cost for testing ranges from $10 for one specific contaminant to $400 for packages.

How about water filters? You can purchase water filters tested by the Water Quality Association (WQA) 4151 Naperville Road, Lisle, Illinois 60532. (Note: there are three basic water filters: carafe, faucet, and reverse osmosis systems.)

Chapter 7

RADICAL PROSTATECTOMY MANAGING LOCALIZED PROSTATE CANCER

Stanley Brosman MD

INTRODUCTION:

There are multiple options and strategies for managing localized prostate cancer. Surgical removal of the prostate represents the first therapy used for this disease and represents the standard by which all other forms of therapy are measured. In 1891, a frontier doctor, George Goodfellow performed the first known prostatectomy in Tucson, Arizona. This surgery was done by making an incision through the skin on top of the rectum and is referred to as a perineal prostatectomy. Although he later worked in Los Angeles for many years, he traveled throughout the country teaching this operation to many surgeons including the new chief of urology at Johns Hopkins, Dr Hugh Young. Young modified the procedure and published the first paper about this surgery in 1904. It was not until 1947 that an English surgeon, Terrence Millin, reported on the retropubic approach that became the predominant method for removing the prostate.

Prior to 1982, only 7% of men diagnosed with prostate cancer were considered to be candidates for this surgery, and only a fraction of these men could be cured. The surgery was dangerous because of the large blood loss, the high risk of incontinence and the certainty of impotency. Then, in 1982, Patrick Walsh, also from Johns Hopkins, described an anatomic, nerve-sparing technique for performing radical prostatectomy. He was able to demonstrate that the nerves responsible for erection could be identified and saved and that this could preserve potency. Dr Walsh also demonstrated that this anatomic technique could preserve continence and reduce blood loss. Although this is a technically demanding procedure and requires a great deal of experience, this is the method that is being used world-wide.

Prior to 1990, the ability to diagnose cancer that was confined to the prostate was limited. More than 75% of the men already had cancer extending beyond the border of the prostate when they were first diagnosed and many of these men had metastatic cancer.

The prostate-specific antigen (PSA) blood test was introduced in 1986 but not widely used until the 1990's. For the first time it became possible to diagnose prostate cancer when it was confined to the prostate. The PSA is not a diagnostic test for prostate cancer but raises the suspicion that it may be present when the PSA is elevated or is rising rapidly. Another major innovation that occurred at the same time was transrectal ultrasonagraphy (TRUS). This not only provided a means to visualize the prostate but to perform more precision biopsies of the prostate.

The combination of the PSA blood test and TRUS with prostate biopsy revolutionized the diagnosis of prostate cancer and enabled more men to be diagnosed when the cancer was still localized. In 2003, 75%-80% of men could be diagnosed when the cancer was still confined to the prostate while 15%-20% had cancer in the vicinity of the prostate. Less than 3% of men are found to have metastatic cancer when they are first diagnosed.

In 2003, more than 200,000 men were diagnosed with prostate cancer and that number is expected to rise to more than 230,000 in 2004. Nearly 30% of these men will be treated with a radical prostatectomy. This translates into more than 60,000 men undergoing surgery each year. It is important to understand the indications or eligibility for this surgery, its complications and the expected outcome.

BENEFITS OF RADICAL PROSTATECTOMY

This procedure is primarily employed in an effort to **cure** the disease but this is dependant upon all of the cancer cells still residing within the prostate. This can be predicted by knowing the PSA, and the grade and stage of the tumor and applying this data into a predictive nomogram such as the Kattan and Partin nomograms. Another benefit of surgery is in a man with cancer but who also has a large prostate which is causing problems with urination. By removing the prostate, both problems can be solved. Surgery is used to treat a recurrence after radiation therapy. This is a difficult procedure resulting in a higher incidence of incontinence and impotency. A third indication is **tumor reduction.** The cancer may not be totally contained within the prostate but removing the prostate removes most of the tumor and additional therapy such as radiation and hormonal therapy can be used to manage the residual disease. This also reduces the incidence of local recurrence.

An important benefit of surgery is the ability to remove the lymph nodes closest to the prostate. This permits an **accurate staging** of the disease. When the pathologist has the opportunity to exam the prostate, the **correct tumor grade** can be established. Nearly 35% of cancers have a higher grade than found on biopsy and another 20% have a lower grade. Removal of the prostate represents the **ultimate biopsy.** With the information obtained by accurate grading and staging of the cancer, predictions can be made about the prospects for long term cure or the need for additional therapy.

In appropriate candidates, the **nerves controlling erection can be preserved.** The best opportunity to maintain erectile function is by performing a nerve-sparing radical prostatectomy. None of the other therapeutic options can preserve these nerves.

Another benefit is the **peace of mind** gained by knowing that the cancer is gone.

CANDIDATES FOR RRP

Men who have a **biologically significant cancer** as defined by a PSA less than 10, a predominantly grade 3 cancer and have an expected life expectancy of more than 10 years are considered to be optimum candidates for surgery. These are the men in whom there is >90% chance of **curing the disease**. Many other men are also candidates for surgery but the need for additional therapy may be necessary.

RISK CATEGORIES

Men can be separated into three major groups according to their PSA, Gleason grade, stage of disease, and the per cent of positive cores obtained at the biopsy. These categories help to predict the risk of cancer recurrence following primary therapy as well as planning an appropriate therapeutic strategy.

Low risk includes the following criteria: PSA <10, Gleason 3/3 or less, Stage T1 or T2a, and fewer than 20% of the biopsy cores with cancer.

Medium risk: PSA 10-20, Gleason 3/4, T2b and 20%-50% positive cores.

High risk: PSA >20, Gleason grade >3/4, Stage T2c-T3 and >50% positive cores.

HOW DOES THE BIOPSY RESULT COMPARE TO THE PATHOLOGY AFTER SURGERY

There is a **poor correlation** in the ability to predict tumor volume based upon the biopsy compared to what is found when the prostate is removed.

A biopsy showing a single 3mm piece of cancer with a Gleason grade of 3/3 which would suggest a very small and insignificant cancer has a **59% chance of having a cancer >0.5cc,** which is a significant cancer. When a single microscopic focus of cancer is found on the biopsy, there is a **92% chance that a visible tumor (>5mm) will be present** when the prostate is removed.

35% of Gleason 3/3 cancers on biopsy will be **upgraded** to 4 or 5 in the RRP specimen and **20%** will be **downgraded.**

RESULTS WITH RRP

The results obtained in eradication of the disease can be separated according to risk category in patients who have only had radical prostatectomy. These results are predicted for an individual who has no additional therapy.

Low risk: >90% chance of no detectable cancer at 15 years
Medium risk: 60%-70% chance of no detectable cancer at 15 years
High risk: 10%-20% chance of undetectable cancer at 15 years.

POTENTIAL COMPLICATIONS ASSOCIATED WITH RRP

Erectile dysfunction.
The ability to maintain erectile function following RRP is dependant on the performance of a nerve-sparing surgery, age, general health, current status of erectile function, concurrent medications and the sexual partner. Even though erections may be attainable, there is no ejaculation since there is no prostate but the feeling of orgasm is retained.

In men under the age of 60, there is a 75%-90% chance of obtaining a good sexual function within one year of surgery. In men between the ages of 60-70, there is a 35%-50% chance of having good erections. In men >70 there is less than a 15% chance of regaining sexual function.

Men who have had nerve-sparing surgery will often benefit from the use of Viagra or with one of the newer agents, Levitra or Cialis. These latter agents have also been shown to be beneficial for men who have not had nerve-sparing surgery. Men start taking one of these medications within a few weeks following surgery. Other options in management include self injection with several types of agents, a vacuum device or the placement of a penile prosthesis.

The loss of the ability to have erections in a man who has enjoyed an active sexual life is a serious quality of life issue. This is a subject that should be discussed prior to surgery and following surgery, therapy should be initiated to restore sexual function as soon as possible.

Incontinence.

Continence has been defined as having to wear no pads or the occasional use of a pad which is only slightly damp one year following surgery. Having to wear one or more pads daily has been found to adversely effect the quality of life for most men.

The ability to attain continence is dependant upon age, general health and muscle tone. Men < 60 years old have a **90%-98% chance of achieving full continence**, those 60-70 years of age have an 85%-90% chance of being continent while those men >70 have only a **70%-75%** chance of attaining full continence.

The various **methods to manage incontinence** following surgery depend on the severity of the problem. Men with mild incontinence can be improved with pelvic floor exercises. Those with moderate to severe incontinence may benefit from collagen injections into the urethra, the placement of an artificial sphincter, a pelvic sling procedure or electrical stimulation of the muscles.

LAPAROSCOPIC RRP

In the past few years there have been remarkable achievements in converting the standard RRP done with a lower abdominal incision into a procedure that can be performed laparoscopically. This technique utilizes the placement of instruments into the lower abdomen through small incisions. The procedure is done using a camera which transmits the image of the surgical field onto a monitor which is viewed by the surgeon. One laparoscopic method utilizes a robot which handles the instruments while the surgeon transmits instructions via a computer keyboard. These laparoscopic techniques are likely to replace the standard surgery in the next 5-10 years.

One of the important questions about laparoscopic surgery is whether or not this is as good a cancer operation as the standard technique. Guillonneau and colleages in Paris, who were one of the developers of laparoscopic RRP, compared the clinical results in 1,000 patients treated with laparoscopic surgery to those have the conventional surgery and found no difference in outcomes. **Laparoscopic RRP is just as good in eliminating the cancer as standard RRP**

In their first 200 patients, Menon and colleagues in Detroit reported that their average operative time for doing the robot assisted laparoscopic procedure was **160 minutes** which is similar to the time it takes to perform the standard surgery. Their **average blood loss was 153cc** which is much less than occurs in the standard surgery and they had to give no transfusions. On a scale of 1 to 10, the average pain score on the first post-operative day was 3. An undetectable PSA was found in 92% of their patients at 6 months following surgery. The **catheter was removed in 7 or fewer days** in all of the patients and **93% were discharged from the hospital within 24 hours.**

Menon also reported that in men less than 60 years of age, 25% were able to achieve erections and be sexually active within 3 months and **at 6 months 82% were sexually active** and 64% of these men did not need any sexual aids. In men over the age of 60, 10% were sexually active at 3 months and 38% were active at 6 months. In men followed for one year, these numbers have doubled.

Continence is achieved more rapidly following laparoscopic RRP. At 3 months, Menon reported that 75% of the men no longer used a pad and **at 6 months 96% did not use any pads.**

NEOADJUVANT THERAPY

The potential benefits to initiate hormone therapy for 6-9 months prior to surgery have been studied. Every report has shown that there is a decrease in prostate size and the presence of tumor extending beyond the border of the prostate. However, there has been **no improvement in long term survival** in men treated in this manner. Currently there is no justification for employing neoadjuvant hormonal therapy for men in the low risk category. There may be benefit for men in the moderate risk group if the therapy is continued following surgery based upon the pathologist's findings. **Men in the high risk group may benefit** if the hormonal therapy is employed for several years following surgery, which may include the neoadjuvant period. There is ongoing research exploring neoadjuvant chemotherapy used alone and in combination with hormonal therapy for men in the high risk group prior to surgery and afterwards.

ADJUVANT THERAPY

Employing additional therapy following surgery is a serious consideration if there is high grade tumor (4 or 5), a large tumor volume, the surgical margins are positive, there is seminal vesical invasion, or there are lymph node metastases.

The types of adjuvant therapy include radiation, hormonal therapy with testosterone suppression, anti-androgens without testosterone suppression, chemotherapy and combinations of these therapies.

MANAGING A RISING PSA AFTER RRP

The decision as to when and how to treat a man whose PSA is beginning to rise after surgery is a subject of considerable debate. There is no consensus as to the PSA value which is considered to be significant. Some select a value of 0.3, others 0.4 and most agree that a value of 0.5 is significant. Another factor is the time after surgery that the PSA begins to rise. A rise two or more years following surgery tends to suggest that there is a local recurrrence while a PSA which never becomes undetectable or rises shortly after surgery is more likely to represent distant metastases. Another consideration is the rate of rise of the PSA as determined by its doubling time. A PSA doubling time of 12 months or less is significant and would usually indicate that therapy should be initiated.

The therapeutic interventions which can be initiated include radiation, hormonal therapy, chemotherapy or combinations of these treatments.

PLANNING FOR SURGERY

Once you have decided to proceed with surgery, there are preparations to be made. You need to get yourself into good condition, both mentally and physically. Having a strong positive attitude that you have made the right decision for yourself and having the support of family and friends, put you in the right frame of mind to have a successful outcome. It is never too late to begin an exercise program and learn and implement a good nutritional diet. Usually, several weeks elapse between the time of making a decision and the time of surgery. It is helpful to stop smoking and to reduce alcohol intake. You should plan for a recovery period of one month, although you will resume many activities before then. The better condition you are in prior to surgery, the more rapid will be your recovery.

Some surgeons will ask that you donate several pints of your own blood, should a transfusion be necessary. Others recommend blood from the American Red Cross. Family members may donate blood if they match your blood type.

Several days prior to surgery, your surgeon will request some blood tests, an EKG and perhaps a chest X-ray. Your internist is likely to want to examine you as well. It is usually helpful to have your bowels cleaned out prior to surgery. You don't want to have to worry about having a bowel movement during the first few days after surgery.

You will be asked to avoid having anything to eat or drink 6 to 8 hours before the scheduled time of the surgery. Any medications, herbal supplements or anything else that might interfere with blood clotting should be stopped 10 to 14 days before surgery.

The day before surgery, the anesthesiologist will contact you and discuss the type of anesthesia that will be administered. You will be asked about your general health, medications you are taking, allergies and previous experience with anesthesia. You will be asleep during the proceed. Some surgeons prefer an epidural or spinal anesthetic in addition to a general anesthetic.

WHAT TO EXPECT DURING THE HOSPITALIZATION

You should plan to arrive at the hospital two hours before the time of the procedure. The nurse who checks you in will ask you to confirm the intended procedure and request that you sign a hospital consent form. She will ask about allergies, obtain your blood pressure, weight and start an intravenous infusion of salt water into your arm. Any additional testing will be done at this time.

The anesthesiologist will meet with you and discuss the type of anesthesia. This is the time to ask any last minute questions. After giving you some intravenous sedation, you will be moved to the operating room. The initial time you are scheduled for surgery is actually the time the anesthesiologist begins to work. The surgery may not begin for another half-hour.

You will recognize your surgeon, even though he will be wearing a mask, and meet the assistant surgeon. Shortly thereafter, you will be sound asleep. When you awaken, 2-3 hours later, you will be in the recovery room. There will be an intravenous line in your arm, a catheter in your bladder, a drainage exiting from the abdomen to carry away excess serum and fluids that collect from the area of the surgery, and special wrappings on your legs to prevent blood clots. You can expect to remain in the recovery room for 1 to 2 hours before being transferred to your room. This is when your family is allowed to visit.

Later the same day or the next day, you will probably begin to drink small amounts of fluid. The day after surgery, you can expect to start walking with assistance. Although it doesn't seem possible, you are not likely to experience much pain. Pain control is achieved by injecting a long acting pain medicine through the epidural catheter, administering long-acting pain medications or with a system of Patient Controlled Anesthesia in which the patient administers his own medicine when the need arises. As soon as your stomach is comfortably accepting fluids, the intravenous is stopped. On average, patients are ready to leave the hospital 2-3 days after surgery. The drainage tube is usually removed prior to discharge.

The catheter that was placed during surgery goes home with you. It is connected to a bag that is strapped to one leg or to a large bag that can hold several quarts of urine. This is particularly helpful at night. You will be given prescriptions for pain medicine and antibiotics.

AT HOME

You can expect to feel tired and sleep a lot but each day your physical activity can be increased. Avoid lifting objects weighing more than ten pounds or straining especially to have a bowel movement. Stool softeners may be helpful to avoid this problem. You won't feel sick and there is no need to spend large amounts of time in bed. It is permissible to begin walking and going outdoors. You can start taking showers when you get home. Soap and water does not hurt the wound.

If they have not already been removed, the skin staples/sutures will be removed 5 to 7 days later in the doctors office or by a home health care nurse. When you return to the doctor's office, the pathology report will be reviewed and a discussion held regarding the need for any additional therapy. There are post-operative nomograms that can be used to help determine the future outcome.

The catheter will remain anywhere from one to three weeks. It is important that the new connection between the bladder and urethra be well healed before removing the catheter. Following removal of the catheter, you can expect to leak urine. An absorbant pad placed inside jockey underwear is generally sufficient to collect the urine and are easy to change. Most men notice that they begin to be dry at night when they are lying down. Bladder control tends to be better in the morning when the muscles are rested and gets worse as the day goes on and the muscles get weaker. It often takes several months before bladder control is good enough to give up the pads although some men still like to wear one - just in case. Pelvic floor exercises help to speed up the recovery. Performing repetitions in which the pelvic floor is tightened for several seconds and then relaxed is a good exercise to do during the day.

Everyone is eager to know their PSA result but in the first month this test usually has little meaning upon which to make treatment decisions. Repetitive testing after the first month can be expected.

You can resume your regular diet but should avoid foods that are likely to produce 'gas'. One of the most common complaints after surgery are 'gas pains'. It takes a few weeks before the intestines resume their normal function.

You should consult with your doctor before starting to drive or beginning an active exercise program.

CONCLUSION

We are at a point in managing prostate cancer where we can give good advice to patients about the ability of surgery to eradicate their cancer. Our goal is to eliminate the cancer with a minimum of side-effects so that every man can maintain a high quality of life. Although surgery offers many benefits, it is not the appropriate option for every man. It is incumbent for each man and his physicians to work together in order to select the most appropriate therapy.

Chapter 8

RADIATION THERAPY IN THE MANAGEMENT OF PROSTATE CANCER

by Dr. Chris Rose

Because cancer cells are "specialized" to do one thing—to grow and divide—they have discarded or decreased other cellular mechanisms used to produce secretions and to protect cellular integrity. One of the ways that cells protect themselves from environmental insults is the production of enzymes to repair DNA. Because tumors have decreased cellular repair, their cells are more sensitive than normal tissue to a host of environmental toxins. Radiation Therapy uses high energy X-rays or particles (protons, neutrons, or electrons) to kill cancer cells. The two most common forms of radiation are external beam irradiation and brachytherapy (seed irradiation). More cancer cells are killed by any given dose of radiation than normal tissue. This is called "therapeutic gain" and allows us to cure prostate cancer with radiation.

Radiation therapy gives equivalent cure rates as radical prostatectomy for localized prostate cancer. When the tumor has grown beyond the capsule of the gland (so-called stage C or stage III) radiation is used either alone or with testosterone blocking drugsandrogen (male hormone) deprivation totherapy to shrink the cancer and sometimes also effect cure.

I. External Beam Irradiation

The task of the radiation oncologist is to localize the tumor in three dimensions and to plan the treatment to maximize dose to the tumor and minimize radiation incident to the nearby normal tissues—the bladder, the rectum, the heads of the femurs, and the nerves adjacent to the prostate which control sexual function. Before treatment starts, imaging studies (magnetic resonance imaging of the pelvis or computer axial tomography of the pelvis) is done to determine the position of the prostate with respect to the bladder and rectum. The patient is taken into a room with a specialized piece of equipment called a simulator that delivers a "dummy" treatment with diagnostic X-rays. Because the radiation oncologist can visualize the bladder and rectum (which have been filled with iodine containing contrast material) he or she can localize the prostate as a negative image sitting between those two organs. Members of the radiation team then place marks on the patient's skin to serve as a guide for subsequent treatment. Patients are treated five days a week for approximately seven to eight weeks on a Monday through Friday basis.

Recently the revolution in imaging, computer technology, and materials science has allowed for more precise treatment, decreasing significantly the amount of normal tissue that is irradiated as the beam traverses the patient to treat the prostate gland. This method is called conformal radiation. Conformal therapy uses a number of different techniques to shape the beam and miss normal tissues. The simplest technique is called multi-field, static co-planar irradiation. That is, the multiple converging beams of radiation lie in a single plane. First, an immobilization device is custom made for each patient, and the patient undergoes a CT scan in the treatment position. A series of CT scan slices are produced, and the slices are "stacked up" to produce a virtual tumor volume in the treatment planning computer. The radiation oncologist and physicist together choose the angles that will optimally conform to the target. Beam apertures are created which closely approximate the shape of the tumor in the particular beam orientation. A low melting point alloy metal called Cerrobend, or Wood's metal, is used to create a physical aperture which blocks radiation except within the area of treatment. Conventional four field prostate or pelvic treatment is a simple example of this class of conformal therapy.

Approximately ten fifteen years ago, radiation therapy equipment manufacturers began development of an automatic beam-shaping device called a multi-leaf collimator (MLC). This device consists of a number of tungsten "fingers" or "leaves" which project into the primary beam to create any arbitrary aperture shape that would be required. Measurements performed on our machine and in many other institutions that have adopted this technique have shown that the accuracy of blocking with the MLC is about 2 or 3 times more precise than that produced by Cerrobend. However, Cerrobend blocking is preferable under certain circumstances.

Delivering non-coplanar therapy is much more complicated than coplanar therapy. The treatment planning computer must calculate doses along every ray of every beam, and calculate dose delivered to each volume element in the tumor (called "voxels") both from the primary beam and from dose that is scattered into the voxels from adjacent voxels. Computer planning times are increased by 50-100 times depending upon the dose calculation model employed. When the radiation physicist believes that extreme accuracy is required, a special dose calculation model called "the Monte Carlo method" is employed. In this case, the effects of billions of single photons sent down each beam path are summated together in the computer model of the treatment. With the fastest supercomputer, the calculation may take a few minutes. With standard Intel Pentium III chips the calculation may take as long as one day. Since automatic plan comparison is still in its infancy, plan optimization may take as long as one week. Specialized calculation chips developed for the national physics laboratories are being declassified and made available for medical research. Also, another method called "parallel processing" will allow the network of computers used for routine administrative purposes in the radiation therapy department to break up a calculation into smaller pieces, and have the administrative network calculate over an hour at night what would take days for a single workstation. Over the past year, a number of the commercial treatment planning computer companies have incorporated Monte Carlo dose transport equations into their computer models. Physics groups associated with radiation oncology departments are assessing the improvement in calculation accuracy and are determining when Monte Carlo is appropriate. For prostate cancer, the improvements in dose accuracy (on the order of 3-5%) may not be worth the increase in computational time or expense. However for the newest form of radiation delivery (IMRT—see below), Monte Carlo methods may eventually become routine.

The latest development in external beam delivery for prostate cancer is called Intensity Modulated Radiation Therapy or IMRT. With conventional radiation, great care is taken to have the beams which enter the patient be as homogeneous as possible. By tending to make the beam orientations symmetric, the dose at the point of intersection is made relatively homogeneous as well. However, it may be desirable to deliver the radiation in a manner that produces irregular shapes and volumes of radiation dose. For example, if a tumor is wrapped around sensitive normal structures (e.g., the prostate, which is draped around the rectum) the tumor bearing volume can be treated without injuring the centrally located normal tissue. In order to perform IMRT, the MLC is utilized in what is called the dynamic mode. By moving the leaves while the beam is turned on, portions of the treatment field which are uncovered for the entire treatment will receive the full dose, while other portions which are totally covered will receive no dose. Thus, the entire dynamic range of doses can be produced in a single field, creating an extremely inhomogeneous beam necessary for IMRT. The technical requirements for IMRT are prodigious: one must assure that the leaves move in a precise manner, that the dose rate of the linear accelerator creating the beam is stable, and that the beam orientations are correct. All of this information must be monitored in real-time and the linear accelerator must be able to be turned on and off rapidly if errors occur. Radiation oncology departments are implementing IMRT in a series of discrete advances to gain experience in what is the most advanced technique of radiation therapy delivery. As of this writing there is only very limited published experience in the use of IMRT in prostate cancer. However it does appear to be safe and doses far in excess of what can be produced for conventional four-field treatment can be delivered. A number of points seem incontrovertible: a) patients treated with IMRT seem to have less rectal discomfort and possibly less bladder side-effects, b) patients can be taken to higher doses than with either conventional or conformal irradiation.

The group at Memorial Sloan Kettering has experimented with doses in excess of 8500 cGy. The issue of what is the highest appropriate dose for patients with different risk factors (e.g., PSA level, Gleason Grade, digital rectal exam stage) remains controversial. Dr. Zelefsky from Memorial has recently compared his experience with IMRT at doses in the range of 8100-8600 cGy to patients treated at his institution with lower doses and conformal radiation. The degree of side effects is less and with a median follow-up time of approximately three years, the PSA control rates appear 10-15% higher. Other published reports from a number of academic centers have shown that doses greater than 7200 cGy result in higher cure rates than for conventional doses. Articles just published suggest that there is yet another break point with even better cure rates at 7800 cGy or higher. We will need to wait a few more years before we are sure that the chronic side effects are not increased and that the PSA control is durable.

Over the past year, published reports from a number of academic centers have shown that doses greater than 7200 cGy result in higher cure rates than for conventional doses. Articles just published suggest that there is yet another break point with even better cure rates at 7800 cGy or higher. For the past three years, limited numbers of patients are receiving even higher doses, in the range of 8100-8600 cGy. We will have to wait a few years longer to find out if these very high doses increase the cure rate even more, or whether they merely increased toxicity.

II. Brachytherapy

Shortly after the discovery of X-rays and radium at the end of the last century, physicians began to explore how these modalities might improve survival and decrease side effects caused by radical surgery.

Within two years of its purification Madame Curie gave a supply of radium to a Swiss physician, and a patient with carcinoma of the larynx was treated and apparently cured. Dr. Benjamin Barringer, chief of urology at what is now Memorial Sloan Kettering Cancer Center (MSKCC) espoused the use of radium needles for prostate cancer in 1917.

The initial prostate implants were performed under direct visualization by the surgeon and the radiation oncologist. Unfortunately, the distribution of radioactivity was imprecise and uneven. Long term results with this technique, which was developed in the 1950's, was less than optimal. Furthermore, with the introduction of nerve-sparing prostatectomies as well as the favorable reports of external irradiation, implants fell into disfavor. More recently, the advent of the PSA (prostate specific antigen) test has changed the way physicians are evaluating results of treatment. Since the PSA can rise years before cancer recurrence is detected, many patients we thought were cured with external irradiation or surgery have in fact failed treatment. A rising PSA following treatment is referred to as biochemical failure. This realization, along with new technologies such as the ultrasound and computer assisted tomography that allow better visualization of the prostate gland, has led investigators to rethink the concept of prostate implants.

Modern seed therapy uses a rectal ultrasound probe directed at the prostate, and a plastic template that is placed on the patient's perineum (the area between the scrotum and the rectum). The template guides the implanting needles. This method allowed for the application of radioactive materials into the prostate in a relatively non-invasive manner, and without surgery. The entire radiation dose is given as a single application sparing the patient the typical seven to eight week course of external radiation treatment.

Seed implants are not for every patient with prostate cancer. Treatment decisions are largely based on 3 well-recognized ways to characterize prostate tumors:

1) Stage: This refers to how big the tumor is to the examining finger and whether it extends beyond the capsule of the prostate. This is sometimes called the T system with T1a being the smallest tumors and T3 and T4 being the largest.
2) Grade: This refers to how the cells look under the microscope. The Gleason score is the most widely utilized grading system, with a score of 2 representing the most well behaved tumors and a score of 10, the most aggressive.
3) PSA Level: The PSA (prostate specific antigen) level is a numerical value that reflects the quantity of prostate cancer present. It is usually placed in 1 of 4 groups: 0-4, 4-10, 10-20, and greater than 20.

A urologist by the name of Dr. Alan Partin looked at large numbers of patients with a wide variety of prostate tumors and asked the question, "Can I predict what the tumor will look like after surgery by assessing the stage, grade, and PSA?" In fact, the so-called Partin Tables predict well for the probability that tumors will extend outside of the capsule of the prostate gland, or invade the seminal vesicles or lymph nodes. These findings may require additional treatment following surgery, usually external irradiation. The tables aid in assessing whether a patient is a candidate to receive a seed implant alone, or if it should be combined with either hormone therapy or external irradiation.

When patients have PSA's greater than 10, most radiation oncologists advise at least some supplemental external irradiation. When the PSA is greater than 20 most advise strong consideration for conformal external irradiation alone in lieu of an implant, with or without supplemental hormone therapy. Grade is also an important selection factor. Results with transperineal implants alone are best with Gleason scores of 6 or less. Patients with a Gleason score of 7 can be implanted although the results are inferior. Sometimes physicians advise a lymph node sampling with a Gleason score 7. For patients with a Gleason score 8 or greater, implants alone are strongly discouraged.

The size of the gland is also an important indicator. The sizing is done by transrectal ultrasound, which gives us the height, width, and depth of the gland. The volume in cubic centimeters (cc) is estimated to be 0.55 X height (cm) X width (cm) X depth (cm). As a general rule, patients with glands greater than 60 cc are at risk for having the most lateral portions of the gland "shielded" by the pelvic bones, and thus having portions of the gland underdosed. These patients are advised to have androgen deprivation (hormone therapy) for three months prior to the procedure in order to shrink the gland.

Patients who previously have had a vigorous transurethral prostatectomy (TURP) for benign disease may have no glandular substance to accept the seeds and may not be candidates for an implant. In addition, patients with symptoms of obstruction may be asked to undergo androgen deprivation first to decrease the risk of acute urinary retention following the procedure.

The first step in the process is an outpatient consultation with a radiation oncologist who will work closely with your other physicians. The consultation will include a review of your medical history and a physical examination. Your radiation oncologist will advise you on the suitability of implant therapy based on your PSA, Gleason score, tumor stage and other factors, and may recommend pre-implant hormone therapy for 3 months or a 1 month course of external irradiation prior to the procedure.

The next step is a planning trans-rectal ultrasound (TRUS). A transducer is placed in the rectum and images (slices) of the prostate gland are obtained every 5 mm. On each slice the prostate gland is outlined, as is the bladder and rectum. The radiation oncologist works with the radiation physicist to determine where on each slice the seeds should be placed. The physicist inputs this information into the treatment planning computer, and a series of "dose maps" called "isodose curves" is generated. The treatment is thus, pre-planned. The physicist and radiation oncologist attempt to deliver a dose of 150-160 Gy with Iodine (I-125), and approximately 120 Gy with Palladium (Pd-103). The seeds are placed and spaced in such a way as to minimize the dose to the urethra. This will lessen the potential for side effects. The physicist orders an inventory of seeds from the supplier that correspond to those specified on the treatment plan. If a patient has received hormones for several months prior to procedure, the ultrasound will be repeated and measurements are retaken.

On the day prior to the procedure the patient is given a cleansing enema and a cathartic. He has eaten a low residue diet for a few days prior to the procedure. The patient may have the procedure under general or spinal anesthesia. Some of our physicians use prophylactic antibiotics but the risk of infection with this procedure is very low. The perineum is cleansed with an antiseptic solution and the ultrasound applicator is placed in the rectum. The template is placed on the perineum and the needles are directed into the prostate through the template. Once all the needles are in position, the seeds are placed by means of a device called a "Mick applicator." This instrument "drops" seeds through and along the course of the needles in a 0.5 - 1.0cm spacing. In this manner a well-defined grid approximating the pre-plan is achieved. The patient is monitored after the implant for six to eight hours. As soon as he is able to void and no bleeding is detected, he can go home, usually on the day of the procedure. A few weeks after the procedure the patient will return for x-rays to confirm seed position.

The outcome of the technique is highly operator dependent. While much has been written, there are many subtle "tricks" and techniques that are passed from teacher to student. It is important to make sure that the surgical operators who are doing the technique have a wide experience.

The only way to compare implant results with external radiation and prostatectomy is to look at PSA control. Unfortunately, there are only a few series with long term follow up to make the comparison. Dr. Dattoli from Florida has published 5-year data using Pd-103. His results with patients who have PSA's between 4 and 10 show control rates of approximately 85-90%, equivalent to the results of Dr. Walsh's prostatectomy series from Johns Hopkins University. Dr. Blasko has 8 year results using I -125. He reports an 80% control rate with similar patients, again equivalent to the best prostatectomy data. Data from the Northwest Tumor Institute (NWTI) reported by Dr. Prestige demonstrated that 2% of patients showed residual cancer at follow-up biopsy two or more years post implant. Another 20% showed indeterminate results with cells that might be viable, or might be dying. With longer follow-up, most of the indeterminate biopsies, when repeated, became negative. The rest (78%) had no cancer in their biopsies and are apparently locally controlled.

III. Side Effects of Radiation Therapy

Even though conformal radiation and seed therapy concentrate the dose in the region of the prostate and minimize dose to the surrounding organs, some dose is deposited in those organs. Also the urethra is totally surrounded by prostate tissue and there is no way to spare the urethra while delivering a uniform dose to the surrounding prostate.

A. External Beam Side Effects

Most patients note increased urinary frequency, especially nighttime frequency during the last portion of the radiation treatment. Patients may be up as much as four or five times at night to urinate. A drug that relaxes the bladder base called Flo-Max may be used and is highly effective at decreasing frequency. After radiation, the bladder base heals and frequency is usually decreased, compared with prior to treatment. Incontinence, which is the major significant risk of prostatectomy, is rare, approximately ½-1%. The major risk of radiation is rectal injury. About 2-5% of men may suffer small amounts of rectal bleeding post treatment. Significant rectal bleeding with modern conformal therapy is likewise rare, but it does occur.

Impotence is difficult to quantitate since many men in the age group of those who get this disease have some difficulty with erectile competence any way. However to the best of our ability to quantitate, 30-60% of men may suffer impotence after external radiation. The symptom does not occur immediately and may take months or years to occur. The oral drug Viagra and intra-urethral prostaglandin suppository, MUSE are often helpful in reversing radiation-induced impotence.

B. Brachytherapy Side Effects.

There is a false impression amongst many prospective patients that prostate brachytherapy has fewer side effects than external beam radiation. This perception may not be correct. Nearly all patients suffer some radiation-related prostatitis. This may last several months or longer in 1/2 of the patients. Acute urinary retention (blockage with the inability to urinate requiring a catheter) occurs in less than 5% of patients post procedure. However, urethritis with slow stream and pain occurs in the first week post treatment. Prostatitis with symptoms sufficiently severe to require the use of bladder base relaxing medicines occurs in 30% of patients. Urinary incontinence is rare with a risk is about 1%. Injury to the urethra resulting in scarring and decreased urine flow (stricture) is likewise rare, less than 2%. Many patients will suffer from some radiation proctitis with very mild rectal bleeding, which may be attributed to hemorrhoids. Frank rectal ulceration is rare, again approximately 2-3%. These ulcers always will heal, and there is no risk of fistulas (openings between the bladder and rectum caused by injury due to the implant). Potency loss is the most common permanent side effect of surgery, external radiation, or implant. The data from implants has always been better than external radiation or surgery. This is very difficult data to quantitate because of patient reporting difficulties, the natural course of impotence in the elderly population that has prostate cancer, and poor history taking by physicians. With all of these difficulties acknowledged, for implant and external radiation combined, the rate of impotence is 75% and for implant alone the rate is 20%. Fortunately, the potential remedies for this side effect including the use of intra-urethral prostaglandin (Muse) and the new oral agent Viagra are as effective for implant-associated impotence as they are for external beam associated impotence.

Multi-modal therapy with radiation and androgen deprivation therapy

Although we have made great strides with better target definition by CT scans and higher doses by conformal therapy, IMRT, or seed implants, the undeniable fact is that not every patient can be cured with radiation (or surgery alone). This is because of the well-known predisposition of prostate cancer cells to metastasize (travel) from the prostate to the area around the prostate (extracapsular spread), the adjacent sexual organs (seminal vesicle involvement), the adjacent lymph nodes, and to other distant organs (particularly the bones) via blood-stream (hematogenous) spread. A biostatistician working initially at Baylor College of Medicine and later Memorial Sloan Kettering by the name of Michael Kattan took data similar to that used by Alan Partin to estimate the risk of lymph node or bony spread of prostate cancer. Basically he showed that patients with either Stage C disease, Gleason grade 8-10, or PSA values greater than 20 were at some significant risk of PSA rise and the eventual development of symptomatic bone metastases despite excellent radiation (or surgery). Groups of prostate cancer researchers have investigated the use of hormone blockade in advance of, during and after radiation to increase the chances of PSA control. Over the past five years a European cooperative group and an American group called the Radiation Therapy Oncology Group both showed that hormone treatment for 2-3 years before during and after external beam irradiation was associated with significantly higher PSA control rates for patients in high-risk groups. Currently similar trials are on-going for patients with intermediate risk (PSA 10-20, Gleason 7, Stage B2). Hormone blockade has also been used for patients with bulky glands prior to seed implantation. While the data here is less mature, the same theme seems to be true: testosterone deprivation can improve the results for patients undergoing seed implant with poor prognostic factors. The seed data is quite early and needs to mature before androgen deprivation prior to implantation can be seen to be standard of care.

V. How can you determine if your radiation oncologist can deliver state of the art therapy?

This is perhaps the most frequently asked question that radiation oncologists and other advisors are asked. The most important factor that is associated with a good outcome is treatment volume. If your doctor does many implants or many conformal external treatments, he has probably surmounted the learning curve. While it is a crude rule of thumb, it takes about 100 cases before one can be even a modestly accomplished implanter. Oncologists doing less than one case a week may lose the skills necessary to implant the gland in a homogenous and complete manner. For external therapy, the case numbers can be lower but the physician should have sufficient volume that he or she can follow his patients and pick up toxicity due to systematic mistakes that may not be obvious. Again the rule of thumb of 75-100 patients per year is probably a good guide to comfort with the procedure.

While the availability of a multi-leaf collimator is probably not necessary to do precise external conformal therapy it will speed up treatment deliver by a significant factor. If the therapists do not have to go back into the treatment room between each exposure the treatment time is reduced and patient movement, the big enemy of exacting external treatment, is minimized. Also Cerrobend block slippage on the block tray does not occur when the beam shaping is performed by the MLC.

The availability and evidence for quality assurance for a three-dimensional treatment planning computer is essential for good external therapy. Two-dimensional equipment cannot perform volume rendering of the target and the oncologist cannot visualize the entire tumor and normal tissues to assure treatment completeness. A special method of comparing plans, a dose volume histogram is extremely helpful in plan evaluation. The patient or advocate should ask if this evaluative tool is available and used in the clinic. Frequently only one plan is produced. While this is usually sufficient, if there is a complicated anatomy more than one plan may be constructed and the physician and physicist need a way to numerically compare plans. The DVH does this.

Finally, radiation oncology departments that are accredited by the American College of Radiology have passed rigorous criteria of quality assurance, peer review, and continuing medical education of the department staff. This is a voluntary program and only 15% of the departments in the country have the accreditation. While not a panacea it is probably correct to say that departments with the accreditation are a good place to start when investigating places to get your radiation.

Chapter 9

PERMANENT SEED IMPLANTATION FOR EARLY STAGE PROSTATE CANCER

Peter D. Grimm, D.O. – Seattle Prostate Institute

There are numerous approaches to prostate cancer treatment. In my efforts to help many men and their families deal with this complex disease, I, like most physicians, appreciate the confusion and anxiety that patients experience in trying to decide what to do. The decision is made difficult because the clinical research methods and endpoints on which to base meaningful comparisons between treatments are not universally adopted. There is also an unhelpful level of disagreement, and even discord among specialists. The result is that there are few firm guidelines upon which physicians can advise their patients and upon which patients can make their decisions with great confidence.

When Michael O'Hara came to talk to me about permanent seed implantation as a possible treatment for his prostate cancer, he had with him a thick folder of information. Mike's determination, discipline, and skill in learning about his treatment options illustrated to me why he had won a place on the first US Olympic volleyball team and in the Volleyball Hall of Fame. He had an excellent understanding of each treatment option. He honored me by asking me to contribute a chapter to this book so that other men might benefit as he had from learning more about their disease and their option of permanent seed implantation.

What Are Seed Implants?

Prostate seed implantation falls under the category of "brachytherapy", a form of radiation treatment in which radioactive materials are placed directly into a cancer-affected organ with the intent of destroying the malignancy. Brachytherapy may be thought of as "internal radiation" in contrast to "external beam" treatment in which radiation, produced by a linear accelerator, travels through the body to the tumor.

Prostate seed implantation refers to the placement of tiny radioactive pellets, or seeds, directly into the prostate using needles guided by some type of medical imaging machine (usually ultrasound). The "seeds" are actually small titanium tubes, about the size of a grain of rice, into which is inserted a small amount of radioactive isotope and then sealed. Because the radiation penetrates a very short distance, the seeds are deposited close together in a planned array to cover the entire gland. Typically an implant requires 80-150 seeds depending on the size of the gland.

Iodine125 (I-125) or Palladium103 (Pd-103) are the primary radiation isotopes used for prostate brachytherapy. These isotopes release radiation gradually over a period of 6 to 12 months, after which they become completely inert. Since the titanium tube is non allergenic, the seeds do not have to be removed and can safely remain in the prostate for the rest of the patient's life.

I-125 and Pd 103 emit "low energy" radiation. This means that the radiation travels only a very short distance before being absorbed by tissue. With the correct placement of the seeds, therefore, a high dose of radiation can be given throughout the prostate gland with little exposure to the normal tissue and organs surrounding the prostate.

The doses from seed implantation range from 110 – 145 Gy for I-125 and 100-125Gy for Pd 103. In contrast, the dose to the prostate from external beam radiation (EBRT) is much less and is limited by the tolerance of the adjacent structures. The tolerance doses for EBRT range from 70 – 80 Gy depending on the technique. The ability of permanent seed implantation to deliver higher doses than external beam is the primary rationale for its use in prostate cancer.

What Is the History Of Seed Implants?

The idea of placing radioactive material into the prostate for the treatment of cancer has been entertained since the early 1900's. Modern prostate brachytherapy was initiated in the 1970's at New York's Memorial Sloan Kettering Cancer Center. The technique at that time was to insert the radioactive seeds into the prostate using an open surgical procedure. With this technique, an incision was made in the abdomen to expose the prostate gland. Using only their hands to guide the needles containing the seeds, the physicians inserted the seeds one by one into the prostate gland. (Figure 1)

Without the ability to see inside the prostate, physicians using the open surgical technique could not ensure that the seeds were being placed evenly throughout the gland. The result was that in some areas of the prostate, the seeds would clump together, resulting in hot spots, while in other areas the seeds were spaced too far apart resulting in cold spots, as illustrated in Figure 2. Predictably, these early procedures were only partially successful in curing prostate cancer and the open surgical technique was largely abandoned when the transperineal ultrasound approach became available.

In the early 1980s, Dr. Hans Holm of Denmark began applying the new technology of transrectal ultrasound to seed implantation. Building on Dr Holm's pioneering work, the ultrasound-guided prostate implantation was introduced and improved upon by the Seattle group to the U.S. in 1985. Using a rectal ultrasound, physicians could now see the seed-bearing needles inside the prostate, thereby better enabling them to deposit the seeds evenly throughout the gland, eliminating the need for open surgery. Equally as important, perhaps, was that the placement could be planned carefully before the procedure and the plan customized to the patient. Also by using a template-guiding device attached to the ultrasound, the needles could be inserted accurately into planned targets in the prostate. (Figure 3) This transformed what had been major surgery into a 1-hour outpatient procedure with little discomfort and rapid return to normal activities.

Unlike the open surgical technique, the more precise ultrasound procedure allowed physicians to achieve the even distribution of seeds that was necessary in order for the radiation to have its maximum therapeutic throughout the prostate. (Figure 4)

In the years that followed, physicians and physicists from around the country and around the world have been trained at courses in Seattle, Arizona and Florida. Today, hundreds of centers across the U.S. are performing more than 40,000 seed implants a year.

Who Is A Candidate For A Seed Implant?

Like surgery and external beam radiation, the objective of seed implantation is to cure or eliminate the cancer before it can spread to other parts of the body. The best candidates for seed implant alone are men with early stage cancer in which the tumors are small and confined to the prostate gland and immediate surrounding area. Patients who are considered to have a substantial risk for disease outside the implant volume are considered for external beam radiation and seed implantation.

Is The Cancer Locally Within The Prostate?

Therapeutic options for prostate cancer can be divided into two categories, local and regional. Local treatments, such as surgery, seed implantation or conformal external beam therapy, treat the prostate gland and a small, 5-10 mm, margin. Regional treatment usually refers to the combinations of local treatment with the addition of external beam radiation to the surrounding areas of possible prostatic spread. These regional areas include the seminal vesicles, pelvic lymph nodes and the area immediately outside a local treatment area.

Selecting A Local Or Regional Treatment When considering a local treatment like seed implantation alone, the important question is not whether the tumor is within the prostate but is it within the area of radiation or surgery? Current models such as the Partin tables estimate the risk of disease outside the gland but do not attempt to predict the risk of disease outside the local treatment field. A patient who understands that his risk of disease outside the prostate is 30% is often confused when his physician tells him that he has a 90% chance of the cancer being controlled with a local treatment. It is important to understand why both the patient and the physician can be correct.

Is The Disease Within The Prostate? The Partin tables and other predictive models estimate tumor extent primarily using three pretreatment factors: stage Gleason Grade and Stage. While other factors may be considered, these factors are the most powerful predictors of disease beyond the prostate.

Stage: Tumor stage refers to the palpable or identifiable extent of cancer within or outside the gland. Stage as understood by most studies is a clinical stage, determined by the digital rectal exam, CT and bone scan. Newer staging system incorporate the results of the biopsy or Ultrasound, however the studies to date do not use this and therefore patients should be advised to understand their stage according to the older systems if they are to evaluate results. The extent of the disease on biopsy does not influence the stage in the older staging system and recent studies have demonstrated that the extent of disease on biopsy does not likely influence results. Buyyounouski, Fox Chase ASTRO #2091

Again, physicians often make the mistake of reading the pathology report and then determining the stage from the report. While some newer staging systems include the result of imaging studies such as ultrasound and MRI, the clinical studies to date have not included these in the staging and therefore their use and value in determining a treatment option should be done with caution.

Under the commonly used TNM (Tumor, Nodes, Metastasis) staging system, tumor stage is denoted by a “T” value that ranges from 1- 4 with alphabetic subcategories (e.g., T2a) that further refine the description of the tumor. Stages T1 and T2 indicate early stage disease, that is, cancer that appears to be confined to the prostate. These patients are often candidates for "local" treatment, surgery, conformal external beam radiation, or seed implantation.

Grade: The grade of a cancer is an estimate of the aggressiveness of the cancer with grade 2 being the lowest and grade ten the highest. It is based on a pathologist's examination of the cancer cells found in the biopsy specimen. As there can be several grades of cancers within a tumor, the cells of the most prominent type are scored from 1- 5 and then added to the score of the second most prominent cell type. The Gleason score is therefore a sum of these two cells types and ranges in value from 2 to 10. The higher the Gleason score, the greater the likelihood that the tumor cells are more aggressive and the greater the chance that the cancer will have spread beyond the prostate at the time of diagnosis.

PSA: Found in the blood, PSA (prostate specific antigen) is a substance produced by both normal and cancerous prostate cells. The higher the PSA level, the greater the concern over the possible spread of the cancer. A PSA level less than 10 is usually more reassuring while levels above 20 are more worrisome for disease beyond the gland.

Partin Tables

PSA, Stage and Grade can each be used independently to predict the extent of cancer. However more recently, attempts, such as the Partin tables, have been made to combine the factors to more accurately predict the likelihood of disease within the prostate gland for an individual patient. With this information it is expected that there will be better selection of patients for local or regional treatment. With the Partin tables, patients can insert their PSA, Grade and Stage and determine the risk of disease in the lymph nodes, seminal vesicles and penetration of tumor through the wall or capsule (capsular penetration) of the gland. By a simple addition of the risk of seminal vesicle invasion, lymph node involvement and capsular penetration, patients and their physicians can predict the risk of disease beyond the prostate gland.

Is The Disease Outside The Local (Brachytherapy) Treatment Field?

The fundamental error made by many patients and their physicians in using the Partin tables and other models is to assume that the risk of disease beyond the prostate is equal to the risk of failure from a local therapy. This is not true. While tumor in the seminal vesicles (SV) and the lymph nodes (LN) likely is beyond the prostate and treatment area typically covered by seed implantation, surgery or conformal EBRT, capsular penetration is often within the confines of these treatments.

Why Local Treatment Can Be Successful Despite Capsular Penetration

SV and LN involvement typically are only small components of the overall risk of disease outside the prostate. The majority of disease outside the prostate is by capsular penetration (CP) particularly in early stages. Capsular penetration (CP) does not mean that local treatment will fail. Several excellent pathologic studies after radical prostatectomy have demonstrated that CP, when it has occurred, is often only a few millimeters beyond the border, well within the confines of a brachytherapy, conformal EBRT and surgical margin. The John Hopkins group demonstrated that only 25% of patients with CP failed surgery if the Gleason score was 6 or less and approximately 50% if the Gleason score was 7 or greater. Therefore, a patient with a 28% chance of CP would have only a (0.25 times 28%) or 7% risk of disease outside the local treatment area. If the risk of LN involvement is 1% and 2% risk of SV are added to this risk, the total risk of disease beyond the local treatment field is 10% and a successful local treatment should result in 90% control rate.

Treatment Selection For Brachytherapy: How Is Implant Alone Or Implant Plus External Beam Decided?

As a result of PSA testing and the increasing awareness of the importance of early detection, most prostate cancers are now being diagnosed in the earlier stages when the cancer is within the prostate and immediate surrounding area. The result of implant alone for these patients is very high. The challenge is to predict which patients have disease beyond the implant volume and would likely benefit from the addition of EBRT.

A determination of the probability of disease beyond an implant only field is very helpful as it identifies patients who qualify for an implant and will not likely benefit from external beam radiation and implantation. Clinical results from brachytherapy studies and Partin table analyses have identified patient groups that likely will need only implantation.

Patients with PSA less than 10, Gleason scores 2-6 and T1 T2a diseases are placed in a favorable category. These patients have a low likelihood of disease beyond the implant volume and have an excellent prognosis with implant alone. Other factors, including the number of biopsies, perineural invasion and possibly the results of imaging studies such as MRI are also considered. It is safe to say that in general, these factors are of less significant than the Stage, Grade and PSA. The determination whether to add EBRT is a decision by the individual physician and patient.

Patients with features other than favorable are placed into two categories, intermediate and high risk. Intermediate group patients are defined as having one factor that is unfavorable, either a grade of 7 or higher, a stage of T2C or higher or a PSA greater than 10 ng/ml. These patients should be considered for EBRT and seeds. However, intermediate patients are often only at slightly higher risk of having disease beyond the implant volume and therefore implant alone may be a perfectly suitable option for some patients.

Patients with two unfavorable features (PSA greater than 10, Gleason grade greater than 7 or T2b or higher) fall into the high-risk category. This category of patients is also often referred as an unfavorable group. These patients have a substantial risk of having disease beyond the implant volume and certainly warrant combine EBRT and implant and possible hormonal therapy

Adding Hormone Therapy: Also referred to as "hormone deprivation", "anti-androgen therapy", and "complete hormone blockade", this form of treatment uses prescription medications and injections to lower the levels of testosterone in the blood. Testosterone, the male sex hormone responsible for the development of masculine characteristics, has the effect of promoting the growth of certain prostate cancer cells.

Hormonal therapy works by depriving both the cancerous and non-cancerous prostate of testosterone. Many of the normal and cancer cells require testosterone and they will die without it. There are several approaches to hormonal treatment. Doctors use "neoadjuvant" hormonal therapy refers to the use of hormonal agents before the primary treatment (e.g., seeds, surgery, etc.). "Adjuvant" therapy occurs during or after the primary treatment. Hormonal treatment also varies by the level of intensity with which it is administered. Depending upon the degree to which testosterone suppression is considered medically appropriate, multiple chemical agents can be used simultaneously. Finally, as with many types of medical intervention, hormonal treatment has certain side effects, including hot flashes, loss of sex drive, fatigue, and weight gain to name the more common ones.

Hormonal therapy has been used principally as a life-prolonging treatment for patients with advanced, metastatic prostate cancer. More recently, however, clinical investigators have begun to look into the question of whether or not hormonal therapy has a role in the treatment of early stage cancer. In particular, researchers are trying to determine if the addition of hormonal treatment can increase the efficacy (the long-term survival rate) of the common radiation and surgical treatments for prostate disease.

With respect to brachytherapy, hormonal therapy has been used for many years because of its capacity to shrink prostate tissue. For some men with large prostate glands, a portion of the gland can be lodged behind the pubic arch bones making it difficult, if not impossible, to insert needles into that part of the gland. (Figure 5). With 3-4 months of hormone treatment, however, a prostate gland can shrink by as much as 30-50%, placing the entire gland within reach of the needles (Figure 6), thereby allowing brachytherapy to become a real treatment option for men who would otherwise not have been suitable candidates.

As to the larger issue of improving survival rates, clinical investigators have begun exploring whether or not hormone treatment can have a role to play in improving the cancer control rates, particularly for disease treated with external beam radiation therapy (EBRT). Hormone therapy, with its ability to kill some of the cancer cells, has been demonstrated in some EBRT studies to increase the long-term effectiveness of this type of radiation.

In the case of brachytherapy, the addition of hormonal treatment has not yet been shown to provide a clear benefit in terms of increased long-term cancer control rates. However, the question of a patient's "risk status" may turn out to be an important consideration going forward.

For patients at low risk of having cancer cells outside of the prostate, seeds alone (monotherapy) has become the generally accepted standard of treatment. For these patients, the substantial radiation dose provided by seeds has yielded excellent long-term results and it is unlikely, therefore, that the addition of hormonal therapy will improve survival rates to a significant degree. This is not to say that hormonal therapy has no place in the treatment of low risk disease. Clearly, some patients (and physicians) will derive considerable psychological benefit from the belief that all reasonable steps are being taken to improve the chances for a cancer-free future and in the treatment of cancer, confidence and hope are important contributors to overall patient well being.

However, it is for patients at higher risk of having microscopic cancer cells outside of the prostate that hormonal therapy may hold real promise. In these cases, seeds, in combination with external beam radiation (EBRT) is the accepted standard of care. With combined treatment, the radiation dose delivered by EBRT to the tissue surrounding the prostate is limited to a "tolerance dose" of 45-50Gy in order to minimize radiation damage to the adjacent structures and minimize the side effects commonly associated with external beam therapy. While capable of killing microscopic disease, this tolerance dose level is generally inadequate for larger tumors. Therefore, the rationale for hormonal therapy under a combination treatment protocol has been to reduce the number of cancer cells in the hope that the EBRT component will be more effective. At the Seattle Prostate and other cancer centers around the country, clinical studies are underway to test the value of adding hormone therapy to the treatment of intermediate and high-risk patients receiving both seeds and EBRT.

To date, the addition of hormonal therapy for intermediate risk patients undergoing EBRT and seeds has not improved the cancer control rates as measured by PSA. The addition of hormonal therapy to high risk patients has been shown to have some small benefit, however larger more controlled studies need to be done

The guidelines described above for deciding on when to use seed implants alone or in combination with other therapies have been stated in very broad terms and should not be considered as absolute rules. Clearly, cancer is a complex disease and the array of diagnostic tools and treatment options all have limitations. Moreover, experienced clinicians may differ somewhat in their assessment of patients with similar characteristics. Clinical judgement, patient preferences and tolerances, and many other factors are considered when making decisions regarding treatment. The chances for the best possible outcomes, therefore, are increased when well-informed patients work in close consultation with experienced physicians.

The Seed Implant Procedure

Seed implantation involves three distinct phases: planning the procedure, performing it, and quality assessment.

Procedure Planning: Since the success of an implant depends on the accurate placement of seeds throughout the prostate gland, the first step in the treatment process is to carefully map the prostate to determine the size and shape of the gland. This is accomplished with an ultrasound "volume study", a relatively simple procedure that can be performed in a doctor's office or the outpatient department of a hospital.

To carry out the volume study, an ultrasound probe is inserted into the rectum and moved along the length of the prostate, taking cross-sectional images every few millimeters. The special software built into the ultrasound equipment allows the clinical staff to outline the prostate on each image. (Figure 7) Using these electronic images, the software automatically calculates the volume of the prostate in cubic centimeters. A volume of 60 cc's is generally considered the maximum size for a satisfactory implant to be performed.

The next step in planning an implant is identifying the "target volume", the area that must be covered, or targeted, by radiation. To do this, a radiation oncologist will take each of the volume study images and circle the area that should receive radiation. In general, the target volume will extend beyond the prostate itself to include 2-5 millimeters of tissue surrounding the entire gland. (Figure 8) As capsular penetration can occur even in patients with very early stage disease it is important to include this "prostate margin" in the target volume in order to treat microscopic cancer cells that may have spread to the tissue immediately outside the gland. It is for this same reason that surgeons try to remove an extra layer of tissue (the surgical margin) from around the prostate when performing radical prostatectomies.

Once the "target volume" has been specified on each volume study image, radiation physics personnel use specialized computer software to create a "dosimetry plan" which is a detailed map of the implant that specifies the number, strength and distribution of seeds that will provide the proper dose of radiation to the prescribed area. The result of the planning process is a detailed map describing the needle placement and number of seeds per needle. On average, approximately 100-125 seeds are used in a typical implant procedure.

Performing the Implant: A brachytherapy team of a radiation oncologist, urologist, anesthesiologist and nursing team typically perform the seed implantation as an outpatient procedure. It is usually performed under spinal anesthesia in a surgical suite and usually lasts between 30 and 90 minutes depending on the requirements of a particular case.

In the operating room, patients are positioned on the OR table in the same way that they were for the ultrasound volume study described earlier. The physicians then replicates the printed volume study images on a live ultrasound monitor. (Figure 9) This is a crucial step because the volume study images formed the basis of the dosimetry plan, or map, that determined where the needles should be placed. Once the proper images have been established, the needles are inserted one by one, through the perineum (the area between the anus and scrotum) and into the prostate. The needles are guided to their planned destination by means of a template devise with uniformly spaced holes that correspond to a grid used in the dosimetry plan. (Figure 10) When a needle has been inserted to the correct depth and its position confirmed by ultrasound (Figure 11), the seeds are released into the prostate. At the close of the procedure, ultrasound and fluoroscopy are used to assess the adequacy of the seed distribution in the prostate

(Figure 12) and if any gaps in spacing are discovered, they are corrected using extra seeds that are kept on hand for this purpose.

Quality Assurance During the implant the primary role of the radiation oncologist is to assess the location of the placed seeds and make adjustments as necessary. As mentioned above, the assessment is done by carefully viewing the ultrasound images and fluoroscopy during the procedure. On the day following the implant, or within a month, a pelvic x-ray, chest x-ray, and a CT scan are taken. The pelvic x-ray (Figure 4) provides the implant team with general information about the implant and aids in counting the seeds. The chest x-ray is performed to determine if any seeds were have migrated to the lungs. Seeds can migrate by being deposited in the large veins surrounding the prostate (This occurs occasionally and does not appear to cause any harm to patients.) Finally, a series of CT scans of the prostate is taken at the same 5mm intervals as the earlier ultrasound volume study images.(Figure 13) The corresponding CT and ultrasound images are then used by radiation physics personnel to calculate the radiation dose received by the prostate and surrounding tissue.

What Are The Side Effects And Complications Of Seed Implants?

The most appealing aspects of seed implants are the convenience of a single outpatient treatment, the rapid return to normal activities (usually within 2-3 days), the lack of significant pain or discomfort during and after the procedure, and the relatively low frequency of serious side effects and complications.

Like other approaches to treating prostate cancer, there are likely short term and less likely long-term side effects associated with seed implantation. Urination is the most likely function affected and is result of the irritation from the radiation. As the seeds lose their radioactivity, these urinary symptoms typically disappear. If necessary, they can be treated with a variety of prescription and over-the-counter medications.

Short-Term Side Effects: The first few urinations after seed implantation can be uncomfortable and there may be some blood in the urine.. This pain resolves quickly and the bleeding typically resolves within a few days. In the area where the needles were placed, there also can be some tenderness and bruising. While this causes some discomfort, it seldom requires pain medication other than Tylenol extra strength..

A more significant problem that some patients can face in the first day or weeks following an implant is the need for a temporary urinary catheter. Occasionally, a clot can form in the bladder or the prostate swells to the point where enough pressure is placed on the urethra to block the passage of urine. If the reason is clots in the bladder, the catheter can be removed within several days. If it is caused by the radiation and swelling, it is possible for the catheter is be in place for several weeks. About 1 in 10 patients will need a temporary catheter and the risk is somewhat greater for men with larger prostate glands. The need for long-term catheterization is rare, approximately 1 in 100.

The catheter is generally removed immediately after implantation. Men who require the temporary catheter generally start with an "in-dwelling" catheter, a thin tube that is inserted through the urethra into the bladder allowing continuous drainage into a bag affixed to the thigh. Those few patients who do not regain urinary control after a month or so may switch to a "suprapubic" catheter which is inserted into the bladder through the abdomen. This device is more convenient since it does not require a drainage bag and provides an on/off valve that gives patients control over when urine is released from the bladder, does not require a bag, and keeps the catheter out of the urethra.

Beyond the immediate post-op period and during the first year following treatment, some patients may experience a need to urinate more often (urinary frequency) and can find it difficult to wait when that need arises (urinary urgency). In addition, some men will notice a weaker or slower urinary flow. The intensity and duration of these temporary symptoms will vary from patient to patient and generally wane with time and generally respond to medications.

Long-Term Complications: An attractive feature of seed implants is the low incidence of long-term complications that can have a serious impact on a man's quality of life. Impotence, incontinence, and rectal injury are the primary concerns of men and their families. These risks are common to all forms of prostate cancer treatment, but there is a general sense that they are less likely to occur with seed implantation.

The probability and severity of any complications will vary from one patient to another and an experienced physician will be able to assess these risks for the individual.

Impotence: Impotence after any prostate treatment has been poorly studied. Impotence as usually defined refers to the complete lack of ability to penetrate. According to the American Cancer Society, the loss of sexual function following seed implantation is less than with other forms of treatment. The ACS estimates that, depending on age, 10-30% of men will become impotent as a result of seed implantation compared to 40-60% with external beam radiation and 65-90% with the standard radical surgery. With the "nerve sparing" prostatectomy, the ACS reports impotency rates of 25-30% for men under 60 and 70% for those over 70. At the Seattle Prostate Institute, our experience largely mirrors the ACS findings as illustrated in the following table.

Age	**Total Impotence**
Less than 60	10%
60-70	15%
Above 70	25%

Several points should be kept in mind about impotency and the reported results. Most of the results reflect only the ability to achieve an erection, they rarely discuss the quality of the erection. A man's level of sexual function prior to treatment may have a large impact on his sexual capacity following treatment. In other words, a fully potent 70 year old man is likely to have a greater chance of maintaining sexual function following radiation or surgery than would another 70 year old who had been experiencing firmness or durability issues prior to treatment. In our experience approximately half of the patients who are able to achieve an erection have some loss in durability or firmness. Fortunately, between 70-80% of the time, these patients can benefit from Viagra and other treatments.

Incontinence: Incontinence is often not clearly defined in the papers dealing with this subject. For this discussion about seed implantation, the definition refers to the long-term need for an absorbent pad. After seed implantation a few patients temporarily require the pad because of urgency can result from both radiation and surgical treatment. Long-term incontinence is quite rare following seed implantation and is probably caused by an impairment of the urinary sphincter. In our experience long-term incontinence occurs less than 1% of the time. When it does occur, it tends to be "stress incontinence" in which leakage occurs when a man coughs, sneezes, laughs, etc. and requires only a single daily pad.

Rectal Complications: With patients who have an implant as the only form of treatment, about 2-3% may experience some temporary, painless rectal bleeding. When the implant is combined with external beam radiation, the rate rises to 6%. The onset of rectal bleeding can be anywhere from 6-18 months following treatment and it can last from a few weeks to a few months. In addition, around 2% of patients who undergo both seeds and external beam radiation may experience more severe rectal difficulties. For the most part, however, these can be treated successfully.

Radiation Safety

Mention should be made here about the issue of radiation safety since there are often concerns about whether men are radioactive following an implant and pose a possible danger to those around them.

Implant patients have not been shown to impose a risk to their families or close contacts. As mentioned earlier, seeds emit low-energy radiation that is absorbed by tissue within a very short distance from seed. In addition, the seeds lose some of their energy every day due to the relatively short half-life of the radioactive materials used in their manufacture. For these reasons, most of the radiation from the implant will remain confined to the prostate itself. Nevertheless, it is possible that a small amount of radiation will be found at the surface of the skin at the lower abdomen. Patients, therefore, are urged to follow a few simple precautions in the period immediately following the implant. These include avoiding prolonged, close contact with children under 2 years of age and with pregnant women during the first month or two following treatment.

How Effective Are Seed Implants In Curing Prostate Cancer?

In the field of cancer, the success of any treatment is measured in terms of how long patients survive without a recurrence of the disease. The larger the proportion of patients who survive over the long term, the more successful a given treatment is thought to be.

Among cancer experts, 5 years is the considered to be the first point at which the effectiveness of a prostate cancer treatment can begin to be judged with any confidence. Beyond five years, the trend in terms of survival, positive or negative, takes on increasing significance. Ten years is felt to be necessary to be able to compare different treatment regimens.

Defining Success: Most patients with prostate cancer will live a long time. This is good news for patients, however it makes it difficult to determine the success of a treatment. PSA based results have replaced survival and local control as the most useful end point for defining success. Two PSA endpoints are most often used, an absolute PSA value or PSA Progression Free Survival. An absolute value is an arbitrary value for example, less than 0.5 ng/ml. Progression Free survival is defined as the absence of three consecutive increases in the PSA level following treatment.

Progression Free Survival was chosen by a panel of experts as the most reliable means to evaluate a treatment method and also be able to compare treatments. After surgery, the PSA will fall rapidly to low or nadir levels. After radiation, PSA levels may take several years to reach a nadir or lowest level. Studies which attempt to compare treatments using absolute values often perform the analyses too early. If evaluated too early in a study, patients who are stable or their PSA levels are falling may be considered failures only because their PSA levels have not reached the arbitrary nadir yet. With radiation, the goal is not the reduction of PSA to a certain absolute level. Instead, radiation treatment is successful if the PSA falls to any given level and remains essentially constant at that level. For example, if a man's PSA drops from 8.0 to 2.0 following an implant and remains at 2.0, he is considered a success, or "disease-free". If another man's PSA level falls from 7.0 to 0.5 and remains constant, he is also considered a success. With radiation treatment, patients who maintain low and stable PSA levels for over five years are found likely to have their cancer controlled for the rest of their life.

In contrast, it should be noted that physicians consider surgery to be successful when the PSA level drops to 0.0 following treatment. This is a reasonable expectation since, with early stage disease, all of the cancer should be removed along with the prostate. With radiation, however, cancer cells are not killed immediately. Instead, radiation destroys the mechanisms that allow tumor cells grow and multiply with the effect that the cells weaken and die over time. This is why, following an implant (or external beam radiation), a man will find that his PSA level falls gradually, taking anywhere between 1 and 4 years and sometimes longer to reach its lowest point. In addition, many normal prostate cells will remain viable after radiation and normal cells will produce some PSA. Therefore, the presence of some PSA in the blood following radiation treatment does not indicate failure and should not be a cause for alarm. Again, this outcome is to be expected given the way that radiation works on the structure of tumor cells and the fact that the remaining normal prostate cells will produce PSA as they do in a non-cancerous prostate.

The distinction between the way in which success is defined for surgery and for radiation is important to keep in mind when considering these treatment alternatives. It can help to avoid some of confusion and uncertainty that men and their families can experience when faced with the often bewildering array of facts and opinions regarding the proper choice of treatment.

What the Data Show: Since performing the first ultrasound-guided seed implants in the U.S. in the mid-1980's, the physicians at the Seattle Prostate Institute have carried out approximately 5,000 of these procedures and have patients who have been followed for more than 10 years. As can be seen in the figures below, the results of our research give us confidence that seed implants are capable of curing prostate cancer in the long run and that their effectiveness appears to be equal to that of other forms of treatment.

Figure 14 shows the 9-10 year cure rate for 634 patients who had seed implants with or without the addition of external beam radiation therapy (EBRT). With 85% of patients free of cancer, this overall group has done very well, especially given the fact that it includes patients in every "risk" category, low through high. It is also encouraging to find that the PSA level of a large majority of these patients (almost 75%) has remained at or below 1 ng/ml.

Looking at the results broken down by risk group gives a somewhat clearer understanding of the long-term results of seed implantation. (Figure 15) As might be expected, the low risk group has had the greatest success with a 90% cure rate. As explained earlier, these are the patients who had the least risk of having cancer outside the prostate at the time of diagnosis. Even the intermediate group has done well implant alone with an overall rate of 85%. The high-risk group has had the least success as it would with any form of treatment.

While the Seattle group currently has the largest patient population with the longest follow-up, it is encouraging that research at other brachytherapy centers is beginning to reveal results similar to our findings.

In Conclusion

Given the growing number of approaches to the treatment of prostate cancer, making a choice can be confusing and difficult. The most important predictor of success is finding the cancer in its early stages when it is still confined to the prostate. Thanks to the PSA test, many more men are being diagnosed with early-stage prostate cancer today than was the case a decade ago. When prostate cancer is detected in its earliest stages, seed implantation, like other forms of treatment, is very effective and the chances of cure are very good. For this reason, periodic PSA tests and digital rectal examinations by a physician are very important. This is especially important if a man is over 50, has had a close relative diagnosed with prostate cancer, or is African-American. Research has shown these men to have a significantly higher risk of developing prostate cancer.

When diagnosed with prostate cancer, men should work closely with an experienced physician to select the treatment that they are most comfortable with and they should not hesitate to seek additional medical opinions to help reach a decision.

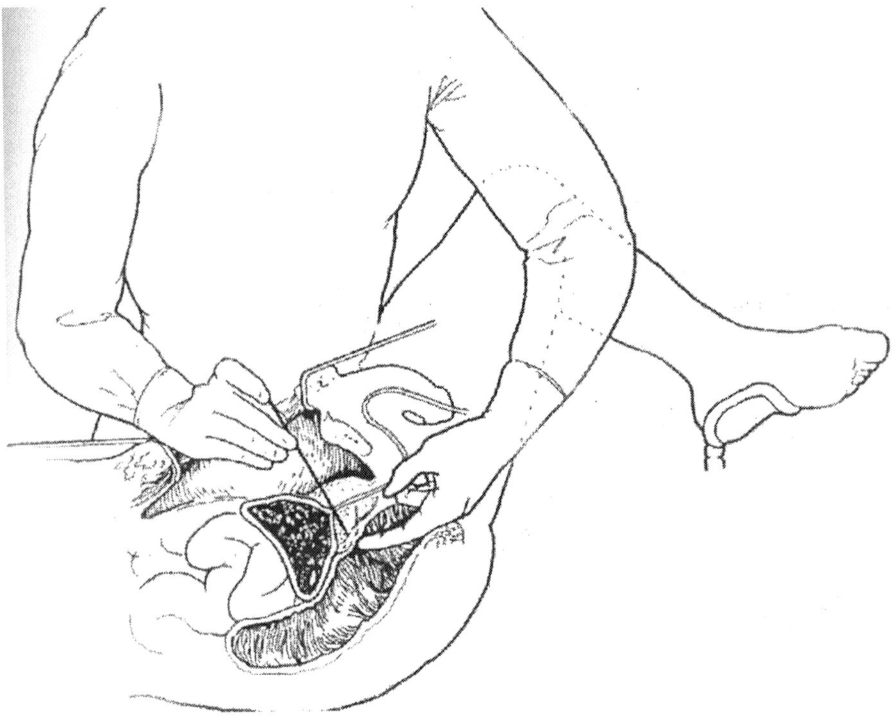

Figure 1

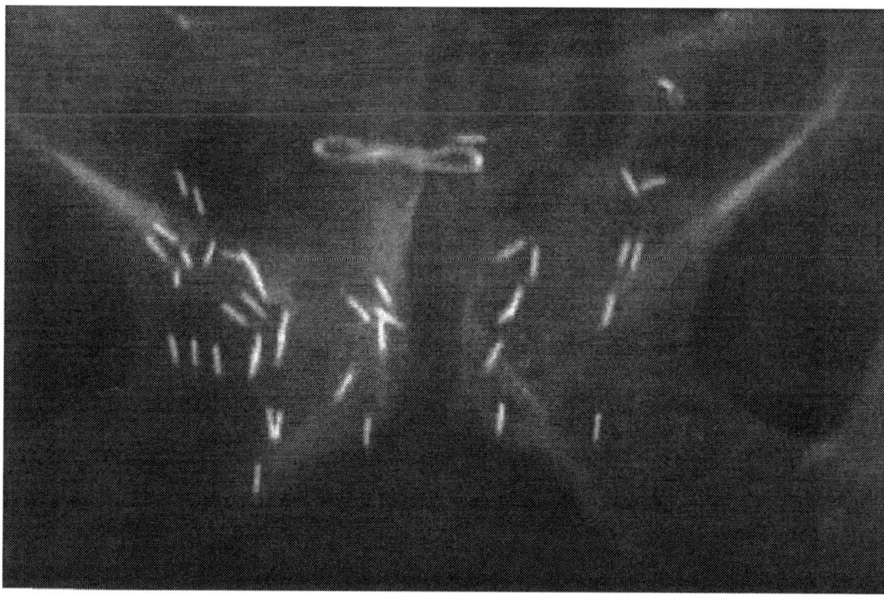

Figure 2

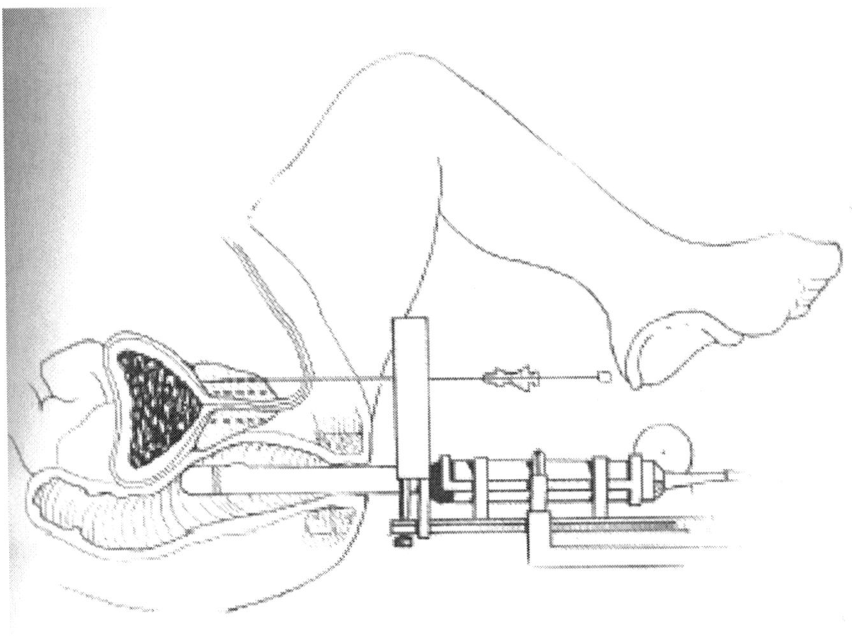

Figure 3

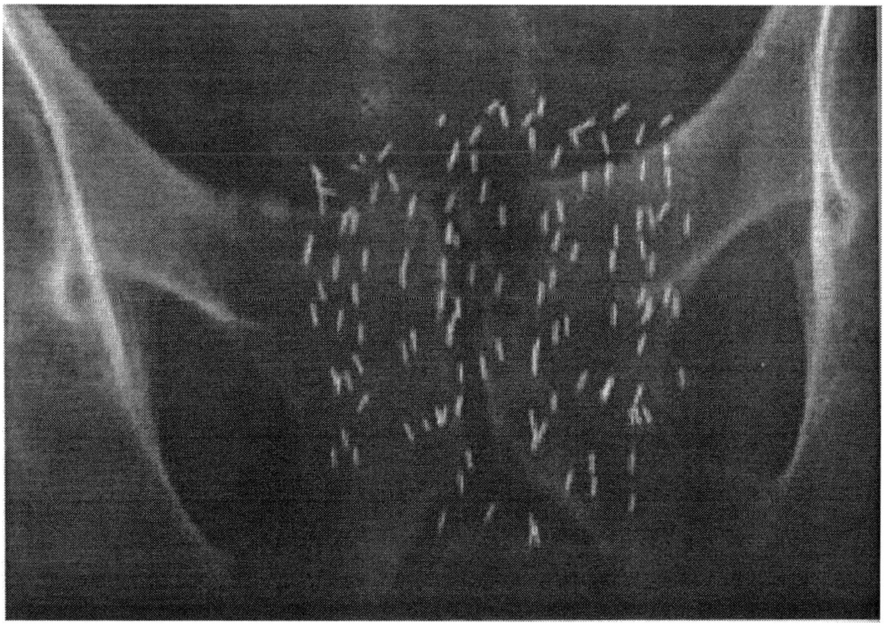

Figure 4

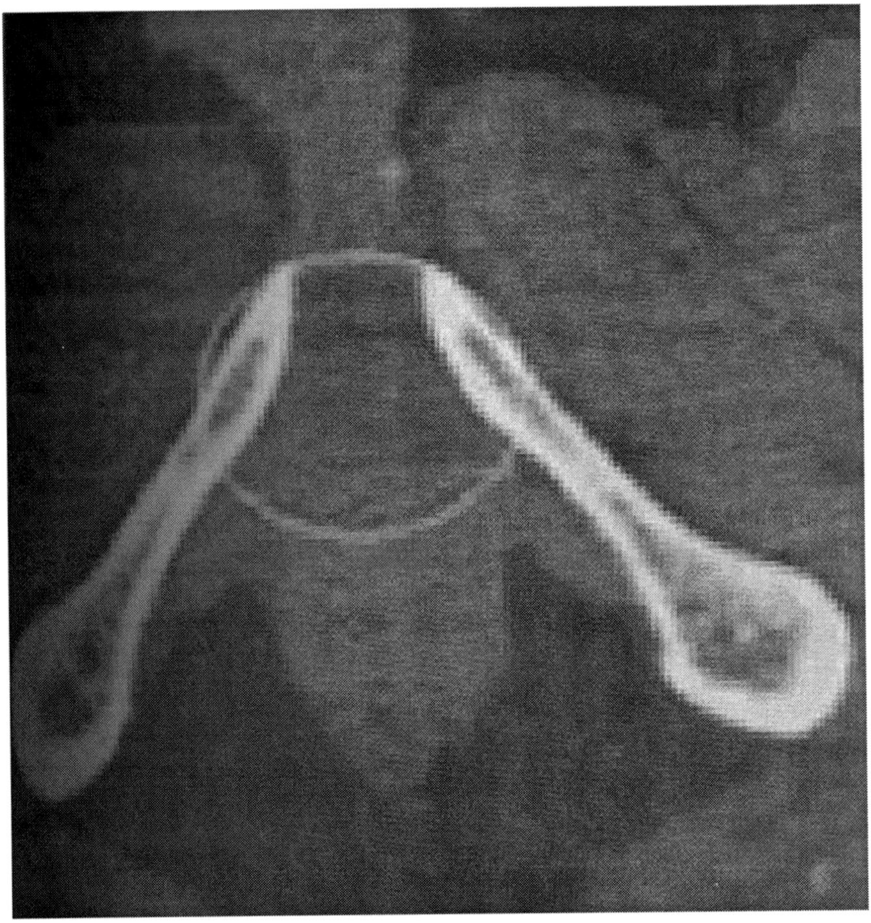

Figure 5

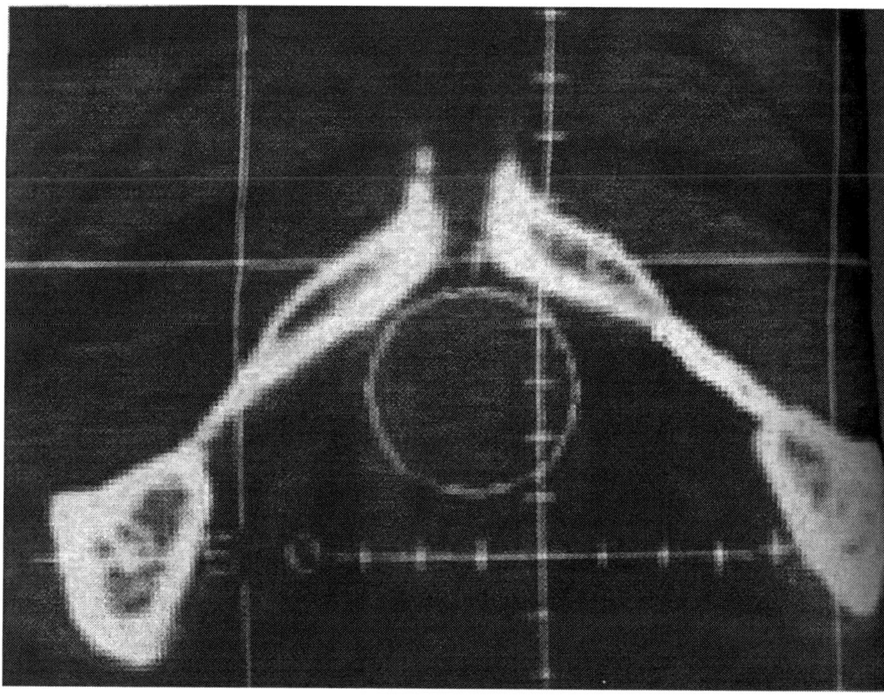

Figure 6

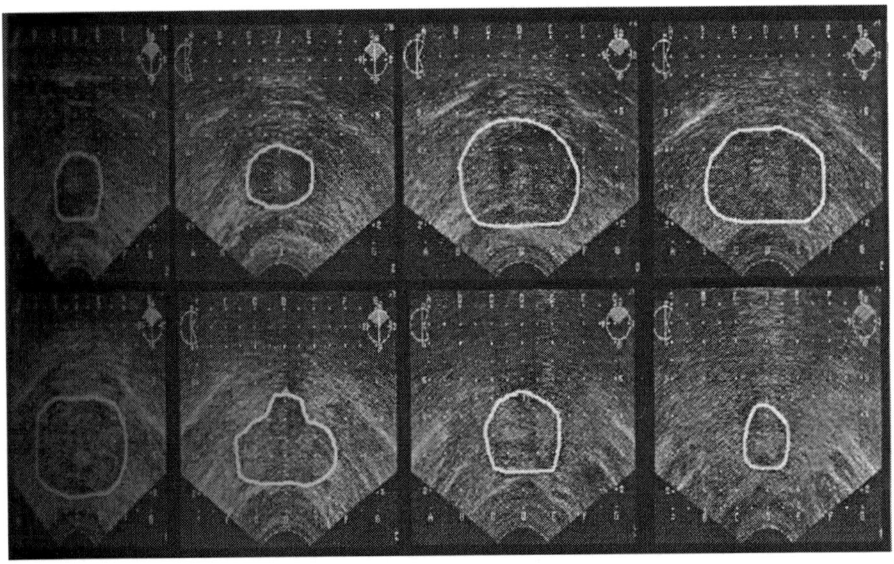

Figure 7

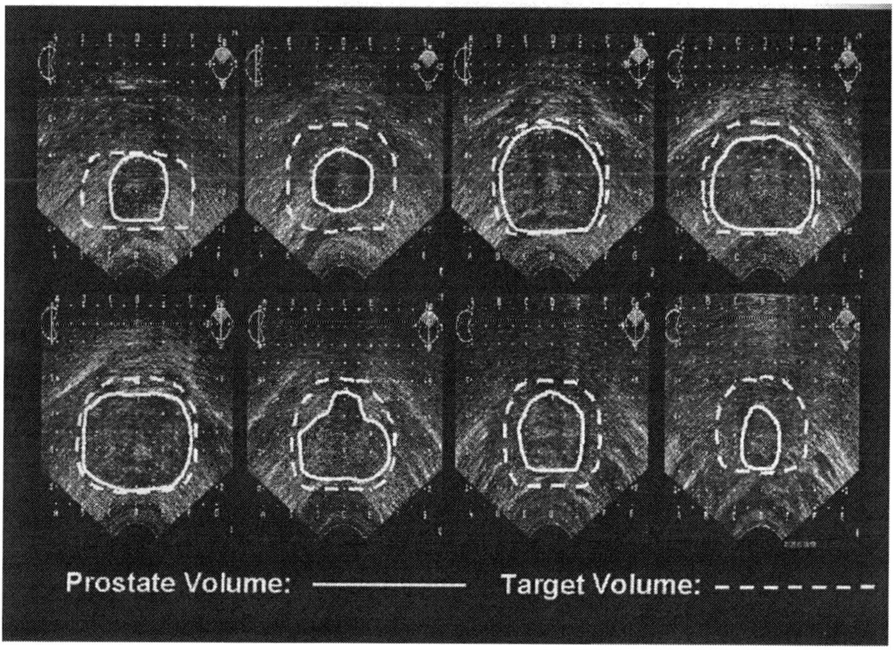

Figure 8

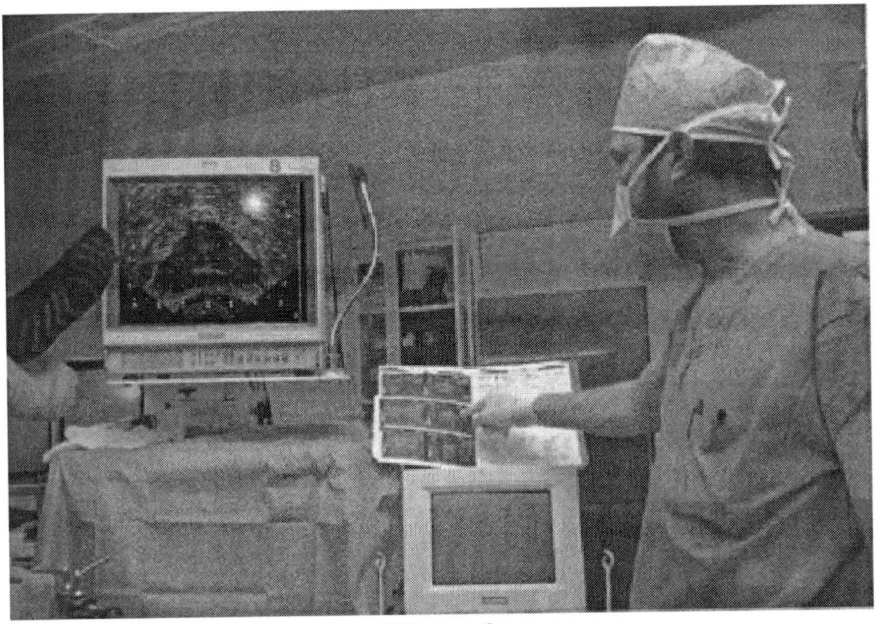

Figure 9

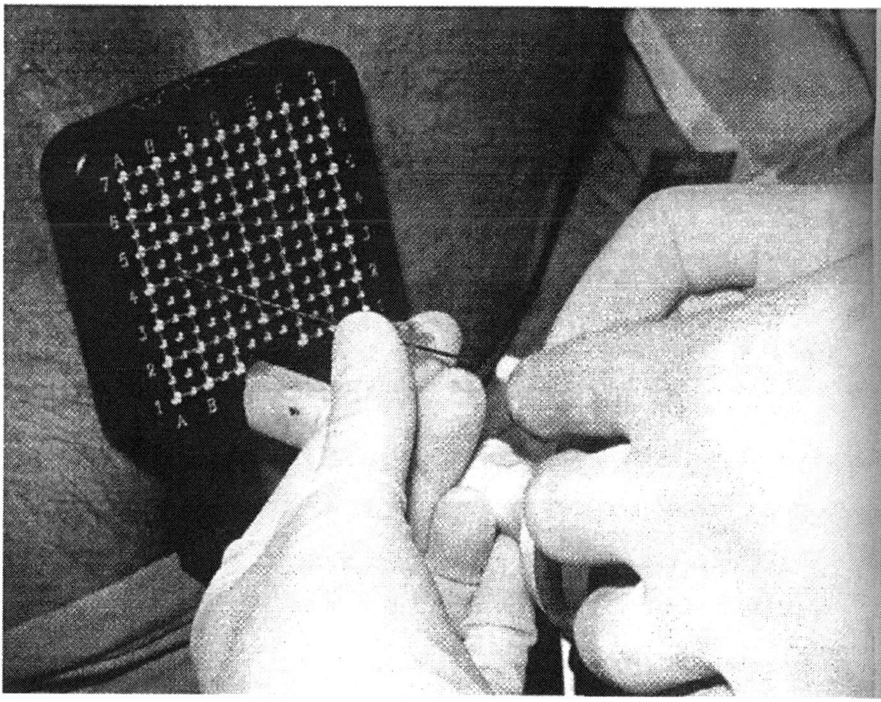

Figure 10

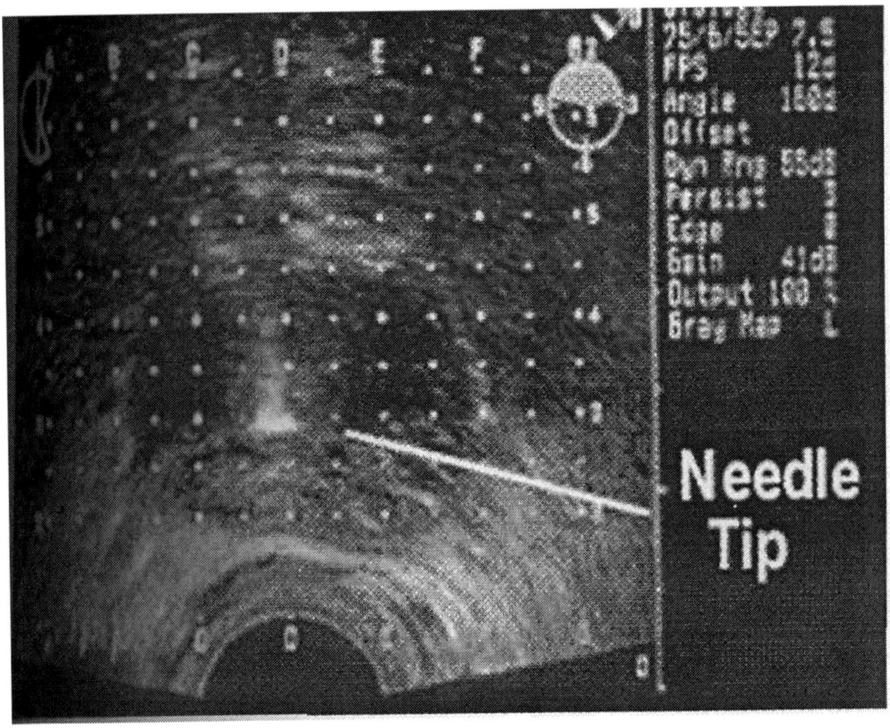

Figure 11

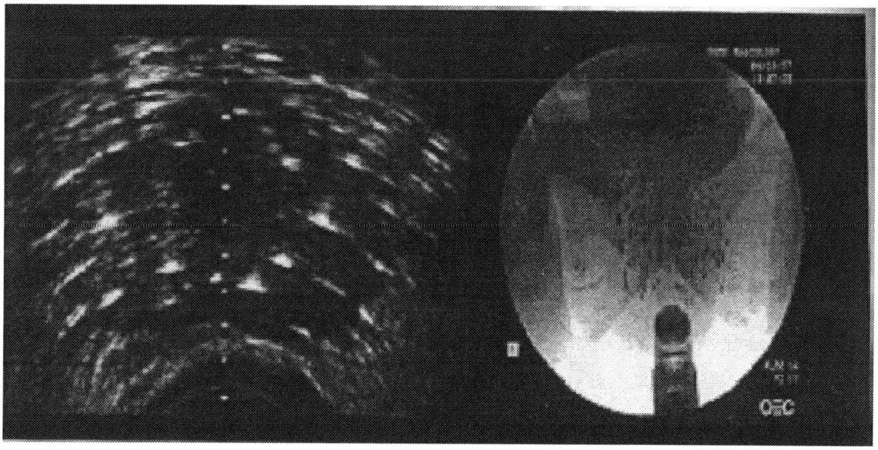

Figure 12

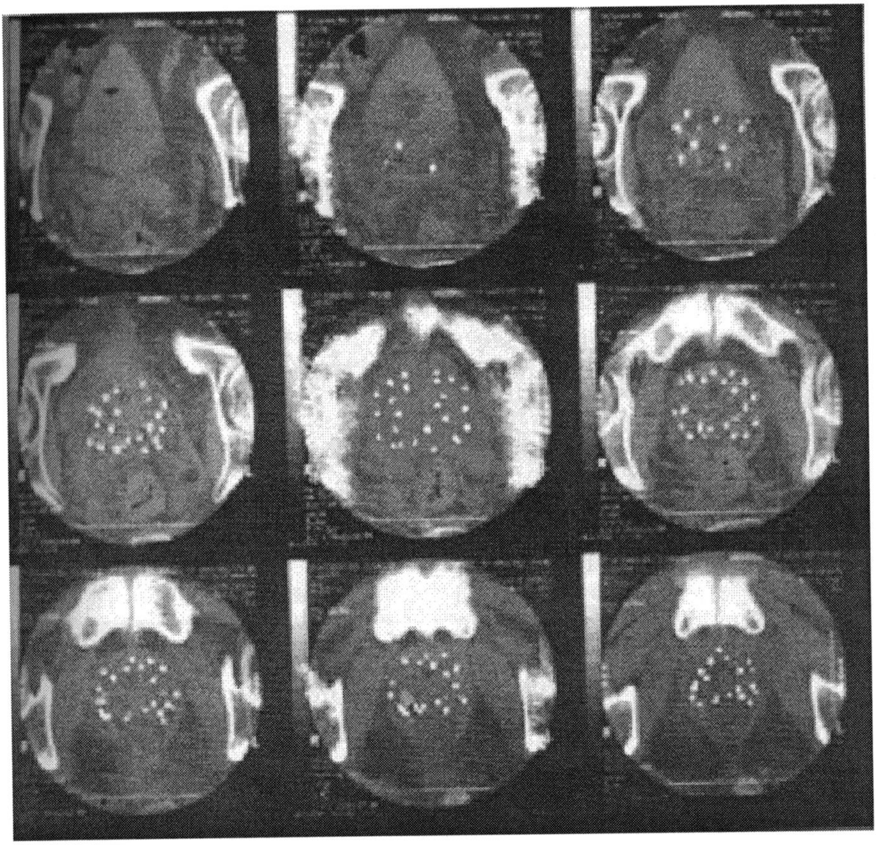

Figure 13

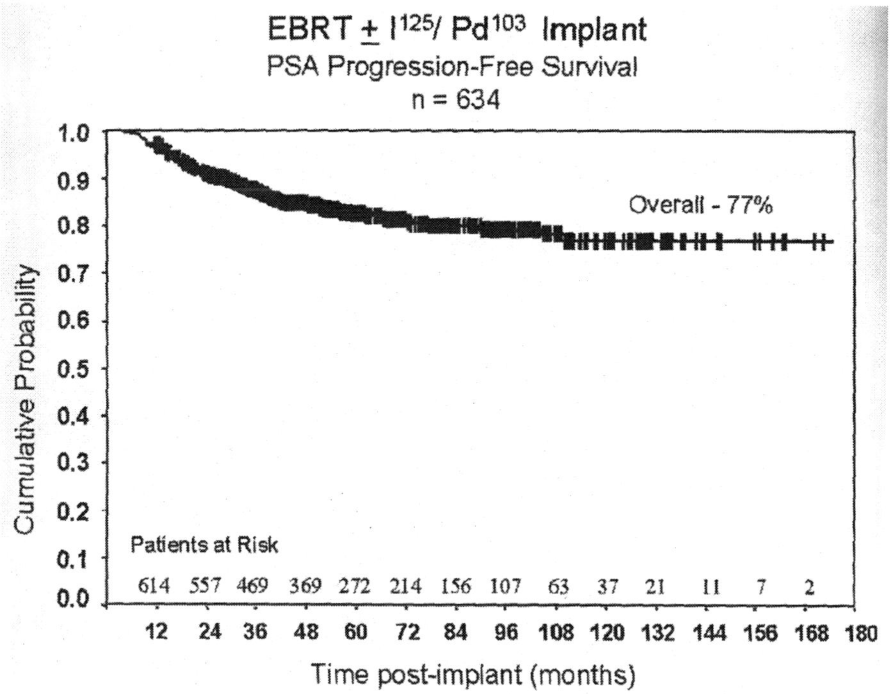
EBRT ± I125/ Pd103 Implant
PSA Progression-Free Survival
n = 634
Overall - 77%
Cumulative Probability
1.0
0.9
0.8
0.7
0.6
0.5
0.4
0.3
0.2
0.1
0.0
Patients at Risk
614 557 469 369 272 214 156 107 63 37 21 11 7 2
12 24 36 48 60 72 84 96 108 120 132 144 156 168 180
Time post-implant (months)

Figure 14

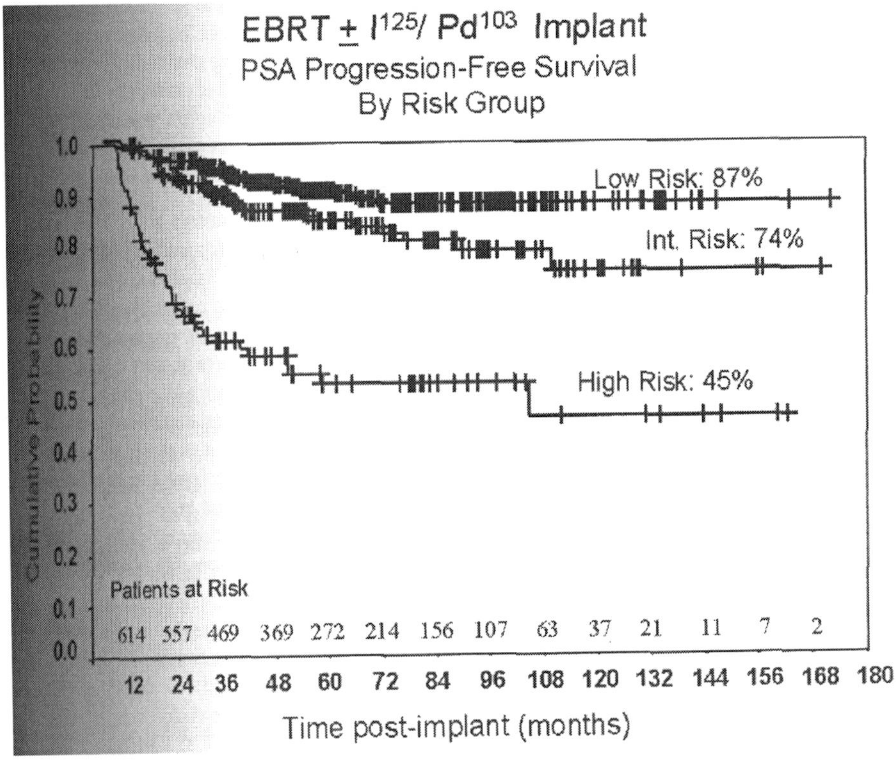
EBRT ± I125/ Pd103 Implant
PSA Progression-Free Survival
By Risk Group
Low Risk: 87%
Int. Risk: 74%
High Risk: 45%
Cumulative Probability
1.0
0.9
0.8
0.7
0.6
0.5
0.4
0.3
0.2
0.1
0.0
Patients at Risk
614 557 469 369 272 214 156 107 63 37 21 11 7 2
12 24 36 48 60 72 84 96 108 120 132 144 156 168 180
Time post-implant (months)

Figure 15

Chapter 10

HIGH DOSE RATE INTERSTITIAL IMPLANT "THE MOST CONFORMAL OF ALL"

Michael L. Steinberg M.D., FACR
Cancer Care Consultant
Santa Monica Cancer Treatment Center
Clinical Professor of Radiation Oncology
UCLA School of Medicine

The radiation therapy treatment options for men with prostate cancer are divided into two categories: external beam radiation, such as three-dimensional conformal radiation therapy or Intensity Modulated Radiation Therapy (**IMRT**), and interstitial implants, also known as Brachytherapy. The best known interstitial implant technique utilizes radioactive iodine, (I125) or palladium (Pd 103) seeds, which are permanently implanted into the prostate. On the other hand, high-dose-rate interstitial implant (HDR), the subject of this chapter, uses a high intensity radioactive iridium (Ir192), in which the implant apparatus is temporarily placed into the prostate and subsequently removed one or two days after the treatment is completed. HDR is an anatomically based application of radiation to the prostate, which is extremely precise and yet technically flexible and forgiving. In many ways, HDR represents the most conformal treatment method of prostate cancer.

DEVELOPMENT OF HDR

Prior to the development of HDR implants of the prostate, a large experience was developed in the use of low-dose-rate Ir192 for the treatment of prostate cancer. The technique involved implantation of hollow needles into the prostate, either under direct visualization at the time of open surgery (laparotomy), or under fluoroscopic, or ultrasound imaging. After completion of the surgical implantation, the needles were hand loaded with "hot" radioactive iridium-192 ribbons. The loaded implant was left in place for approximately two to three days to irradiate the prostate gland. The physician and the nursing staff were by necessity occupationally exposed to a low dose of radiation, as they cared for the patient. This technique allowed for near conformal treatment of prostate cancer. As it was originally devised, it was routinely combined with external radiation therapy and thus, the implant served as a radiation boost to the prostate. This technique was initially used in patients with locally advanced prostate cancer, which involved both lobes of the prostate gland (Stage T2b) or that had extended through the capsule of the prostate (Stage T3). The results of this treatment were superior to conventional external beam radiation therapy in patients with similar locally advanced stage. In our series of over 400 patients a 75% local control rate was achieved, which was superior to conventional external beam radiation therapy, which could only claim a 35% local control rate.

Primarily, as a result of the European radiation safety regulations, which required minimal occupational exposure to radiation for nurses and physicians when caring for radiation oncology patients, equipment was developed to remotely load radiation into patients, with implants. It was most commonly utilized in patients with gynecological implants for cervix and uterine cancer, but later applied to other tumor systems as well. It was called robotically controlled afterloading. Initially, low-dose-rate radiation sources were utilized. However, with time high-dose-rate iridium-192 sources were developed and were used, which shortened treatment time from days to minutes. A large experience with HDR and the treatment of GYN tumors was developed. In the late 1980's the HDR technique was applied to the treatment of prostate cancer.

THE HDR TECHNIQUE FOR THE TREATMENT OF PROSTATE CANCER

The HDR treatment begins with the surgical placement of the implant in the operating room under spinal or general anesthesia by a surgical team, which includes a radiation oncologist and a urologist. The patient is placed in stirrups with the legs up, in the so called lithotomy position. A special template is used which defines the placement and location of the implant needles. It is placed against the perineum, (the flat area between the inferior aspect of the scrotum and the anus). Hollow needles are placed through the template and implanted into the prostate tissue, utilizing an ultrasound device, which is placed in the rectum to guide the needles (Figure 1, ultrasound/implant). After all the needles are implanted into the prostate (between 12 and 20) the template is sutured in place. Then a cystoscope is used to look inside the bladder, to confirm the location of the implanted needles. A Foley catheter is left in the bladder during the treatment course. The surgical procedure lasts approximately 1½ hours. After the patient recovers from anesthesia, he receives a CT scan in ½ cm slices are through the prostate, the implant, and the surrounding anatomy. The CT scan data is then transferred to special HDR treatment planning computers, which can analyze in three-dimensions the radiation dose to the prostate, and the nearby structures (urethra, bladder, rectum). The prescribed dose of radiation is determined by the radiation oncologist.

The computer determines the amount of time the high intensity Iridium-192 source must dwell at various positions within the implanted needle to create the dosed distribution prescribed the radiation oncologist. The radiation dose can be optimized to conform to the prostate gland and avoid near by critical structures by adjusting the time the sources dwell within the needles. Areas within the prostate gland known to have tumor nodules can be given higher doses by allowing the source to dwell for longer time in those regions. While areas adjacent to critical structures, such as the urethra, can be given lower doses simply by adjusting to shorter dwell times. The state of the art computer system can plan for conformal treatment to the periphery of the prostate gland, while keeping the dose level low to the rectum and bladder. At the same time, the computer can define differential doses inside the gland; lower at the urethra and higher at the tumor nodule. It can be said that the HDR treatment is conformal both inside and out (Figure 2, dosimetry).

After the treatment plan is accepted by the radiation oncologist, the computer controls the robotic mechanism of the HDR afterloading device. Cables are connected from the machine containing the high-dose-rate radioactive source to the hollow needles implanted into the prostate. The radioactive source is delivered to the various needles implanted within the prostate (Figure 3, HDR machine). The radioactive source dwells at the predetermined locations within each needle, as defined by the computer plan, thus, delivering the prescribed treatment to the prostate. This process takes approximately 10 to 15 minutes. The treatment is repeated from one to three times, with a time interval of not less than six hours between each treatment. At this time, our group, as well as others, routinely use a total of three treatment fractions. After the last treatment the implant is removed. Removal of the implant does not require the patient to return to the operating room. There are no radioactive sources left within the patient. Most patients are able to go home within hours of the last treatment.

To complete the total treatment course, the patient receives four to five and a half weeks of external beam radiation therapy to the prostate and periprostatic tissues. The external beam radiation therapy commences one and two weeks after the HDR implant.

RESULTS OF THE HDR TREATMENT

As mentioned before, temporary implants are considered particularly effective in the treatment of locally advanced prostate cancer, where other techniques, such as permanent seed implant and conventional radiation therapy have fallen short. There are a number of published series in the literature, as well as three large unpublished series including our series from Cancer Care Consultants. They show excellent results in terms of local control of the prostate tumor, with minimal short term and long term side effects. It should be noted that there are significant difficulties when comparing treatment results between various prostate cancer treatment methods, due to unequal distribution of prognostic factors that are known to determine outcome among patients. These prognostic factors, that may vary when comparing one study to another include, PSA at presentation, Gleason grade, and clinical stage. That said, results of HDR as a boost for locally advanced prostate cancer appears superior to other treatment methods, such as conventional external beam radiation therapy and permanent seed implants. HDR as a boost treatment for early stage prostate cancer is also equivalent to other radiation treatments for earlier stage disease. In addition, the results achieved are associated with among the lowest complication rates in radiation therapy. HDR is associated with the lowest treatment related complications, related to urethral stricture (usually less than 1%), incontinence, (less than 1% in patients who have not received previous prostate surgery) and rectal problems (less than 1%). The risk of impotence is similar to other radiation therapy treatment methods and is reported in the range of 18 to 40%.

THE ADVANTAGES OF HDR

The primary advantage of the HDR technique is its extraordinary ability to give dose coverage to the entire gland, while at the same time offering the possibility of differential dosing, within the prostate gland. With HDR the dose can be adjusted to spare the urethra within the prostate gland, while at the same time, boosting the dose to tumor nodules elsewhere within the gland. This functionality is unique to the HDR technique.

Yet another advantage of HDR is its ability to safely achieve dose escalation within the prostate, while sparing the adjacent sensitive structures, such as the rectum and bladder. Rectum and bladder doses are routinely less than 60 to 70% of the minimum dose to the prostate. Most important however, while the treatment dose at the periphery of the prostate, greater than 90% of the time achieves 100% of the prescribed dose (n.b. 85% is considered superior with permanent seed implants), significant volumes within the prostate gland achieve doses of greater than 125% to 150% of the prescribed dose. This internal dose escalation translates into increased tumor control, due to the dose response relationship previously noted in discussions of dose escalation with three-dimensional conformal radiation therapy for prostate cancer.

HDR itself offers certain technical advantages, due to the inherent forgiving nature and flexibility of the technique. In contrast, the permanent seed implant techniques where the dose planned is based on an idealization of the anticipated needle placement, the HDR technique allows CT visualization of the actual implant needle location relative to the prostate capsule, prostate base, prostate apex, prostatic urethra, bladder, and rectum. If needle deflection occurs, the computer can adjust the dwell times of the radioactive source, within the needle, to compensate for less than perfect placement. In addition, issues of seed migration and seed loss noted in permanent seed implants are not associated with the HDR technique.

Disadvantages of HDR relative to other treatments include the need for surgery, anesthesia and hospitalization. Also, although there are reports in using HDR alone as complete treatment, the current recommendation combines HDR with external beam radiation therapy for a complete treatment.

SUMMARY

HDR offers a flexible yet conformal and precise technique, to deliver dose escalated radiation therapy to the prostate with among the lowest risk of treatment related complications. The technique is particularly effective in locally advanced tumors of the prostate and excellent results are also observed in early stage disease. In fact, more patients are eligible for HDR implants than permanent seed implants, because it is applicable to early stage as well as advance stage disease. In the quest to achieve increased dose within the prostate, HDR offers the ability to differentially deliver dose to different areas within the gland. It can be said, that HDR is conformal inside and out and may well be the most conformal radiation treatment of all.

Chapter 11

INTENSITY MODULATED RADIATION THERAPY "IMRT" "THE NEW - NEW THING"

Michael L. Steinberg, M.D. FACR
Cancer Care Consultants at
Santa Monica Cancer Treatment Center
Clinical Professor of Radiation Oncology,
UCLA School of Medicine

For the newly diagnosed prostate cancer patient, IMRT represents yet another technological innovation available in the armamentarium for the treatment of prostate cancer. What is IMRT and what does its application mean in terms of improved treatment for prostate cancer? In the following discussion you will learn about the technology which makes IMRT possible, as well as how the application of this technology may improve treatment outcomes in prostate cancer.

IMRT is the most precise treatment planning and treatment delivery system yet devised, to deliver radiation therapy. IMRT takes advantage of the practical aspects of leading edge technology in computer sciences, medical imaging technology, materials engineering, and medical physics. IMRT is the most precise method to deliver radiation dosage to the prostate, without the need for surgical intervention. It represents the next technological progression in external beam radiation therapy management for many tumors, including prostate cancer. IMRT is truly "THE NEW - NEW THING".

To understand the technological advancement of IMRT over other external beam radiation techniques, one must first consider what went before in the application of radiation therapy for the treatment of prostate cancer: conventional radiation therapy and 3D conformal therapy (3D CRT). Conventional radiation was first noted to be effective in the treatment of periprostate cancer in the late 1960's. Utilizing the existing linear accelerator technology at the time, radiation therapy was delivered to the prostate and periprostatic tissues in an effort to eradicate the cancer, while attempting to spare the sensitive surrounding normal tissues from potential untoward effects of the radiation. If it were not necessary to consider the radiation dose tolerance of the surrounding normal structures, such as the rectum and bladder, radiation therapy in high enough dose would eradicate the vast majority of prostate cancers. It turns out, however, that the dose limiting feature in the treatment of prostate cancer with conventional radiation therapy, is the tolerance of the adjacent normal tissues of the bladder and rectum. The dose tolerance for these structures is below the dose which is required to eradicate the prostate cancer, with a high degree of probability. The conventional radiation technique utilized a cross-fire, 4 field box technique, which centered on the prostate, but also included substantial portions of the rectum and bladder within the radiation fields. Due to this fact, the dose of radiation to the prostate was limited to a range not higher than 6,800 to 7,000 centigray.

Although conventional radiation therapy was found to be effective in controlling many prostate cancers, in the late 1980's and the early 1990's, techniques were developed to conform the standard radiation beam to the prostate gland and thus, exclude substantial portions of the dose limiting tissues of the bladder and rectum. The techniques developed, called 3D conformal radiation (3D CRT), utilized CT imaging technology, as well as three-dimensional radiation therapy treatment planning computer programs to develop anatomically shaped radiation beams which conform as much as possible to the shape of the prostate gland, while avoiding the sensitive tissues of the rectum and bladder. Multiple radiation beams (4, 6, or 7), are delivered at various angles, with each beam shaped by beam shaping devices, such as radiation therapy treatment blocks, or multileaf collimators (MLC) to conform the radiation therapy beamed to the prostate target. The beam shape is defined by a 3D computer graphics software, which allows the radiation oncologist to visualize the prostate target via a beam's eye view (BEV) technique. The anticipated benefits of 3D CRT were felt to be decreased treatment toxicity related to the rectum and bladder, as well the possibility that higher "escalated doses" could be utilized to give a higher probability of tumor control.

Although, to date, there is no long term survival advantage attributed to 3D CRT for the treatment of prostate cancer, clinical trials have established certain facts. First, 3D CRT is associated with less acute side effects of treatment related to bladder irritation, rectal bleeding and diarrhea. Second, 3D CRT has less long term "GI" side effects, such as chronic rectal bleeding. And third, dose escalation of 10 to 20% is possible, without increasing toxicity to adjacent normal tissues and that dose escalation results in improved biochemical disease free survival as measured by lack of 3 consecutive rises in PSA.

With all the benefits of 3D CRT, the planning techniques have certain shortcomings. 3D CRT planning utilizes a trial and error methodology. The radiation oncologist and the medical physicist define a treatment technique and use the computer to show the dose the prostate receives by utilizing this predetermined array of treatment fields. If the dose is not acceptable, alternative radiation fields, or beam modification devices are used in an effort to optimize the dose. This planning technique is called "forward planning". Simply put, forward planning takes beam arrangements and beam shaping modifications as defined by the radiation oncologist and shows what those arrangements and modifications yield in terms of dose to the treatment volume. The trial and error process of forward planning at times must be repeated to obtain optimal dose distribution. Sometimes, optimal dose distributions cannot be achieved, particularly when the targeted structure has highly irregular shapes, with a combination of convex and concave contours (like many prostate glands). Until now, 3D CRT BEV forward planning represented state of the art radiation therapy planning and delivering.

THE IMRT ADVANTAGE

IMRT achieves unprecedented conformity of the radiation dose, by applying two complex concepts.

1. Inverse Treatment Planning
2. Modulation of the radiation beam, during treatment to change the intensity of the radiation from moment to moment, during the treatment delivery.

INVERSE TREATMENT PLANNING

In the case of IMRT, the trial and error method of forward planning is replaced by a treatment planning process that allows the radiation oncologist to precisely define the dose to the targeted anatomy (in this case the prostate). In addition, the radiation oncologist can designate areas where the radiation dose is not desired, such as to the sensitive structures of the rectum and bladder and therefore limit the dose to those areas. In fact, inverse planning, together with modulation of the radiation therapy beam, can create radiation dose distributions in almost any conceivable pattern.

INTENSITY MODULATION OF THE RADIATION THERAPY BEAM

The second crucial concept of IMRT is modulation of the intensity or strength of the treatment beam, which is varied across the treatment target. To accomplish this, the treatment beam is divided into a multitude of pencil sized beamlets. Each beamlet can, in turn, be adjusted or modulated as to its intensity, with some beamlets shining on the target for longer periods of time or with a stronger intensity. It is like using hundreds of flashlights, each with a different low level of brightness, shining on an object in a dark room. When the flashlights are placed appropriately, the object will be lit, but the surroundings in the room will remain relatively dark. With IMRT, we start with a target, which for the sake of this discussion is the prostate, deep inside the body. The IMRT inverse planning computer system then back projects through the patient's tissue (soft tissue, organs, bone, etc.) and returns to the linear accelerator source, to define a complicated nonuniform radiation exposure plan. With the equipment which is most commonly in use at this time, the Nomos-Peacock System, the delivery of the radiation plan is accomplished by using a multileaf collimator (MLC), which is attached to the head of the linear accelerator, between the source of the radiation and the patient. The MLC contains a set of tungsten leaves, which divide the conventional treatment beam into smaller beams or beamlets. As the tungsten leaves move, so does the linear accelerator gantry in an arc-like fashion and thus, the beam is modulated to the specifications of the treatment plan.

DEVELOPMENT OF THE IMRT TREATMENT PLAN

The treatment planning process begins in the same way 3D CRT does, with a treatment planning CT scan of the patient immobilized in the treatment position. Anywhere from 35 to 60 CT scan slices are transferred to the IMRT planning computer. The radiation oncologist designates the target volume (the prostate) and the dose that the target volume is to receive. In addition, the radiation oncologist defines maximum tolerance doses to the nearby critical structures, such as the rectum, bladder, and the femoral heads. The computer takes all these specifications into account to derive a treatment plan. Also, the computer solves conflicts between specifications of high dose areas (the target volume) and low dose areas, (the nearby sensitive tissues), and also takes into consideration uncertainties in the prostates' localization and the prostate movement within the body, by adding margins to the clinical tumor volume (CTV) as designated by the prostate gland, to create the planning tumor volume (PTV).

The computer produces the plan, which designates dose coverage specifically called isodose distributions, in axial, sagittal and coronal views. In addition, a valuable tool for the radiation oncologist and medical physicist is developed by the computer called a Dose Volume

Histogram (DVH). This is a graphic display of the radiation dose versus the volume of the target and the nearby sensitive tissues. If the plan shows the appropriate coverage of the target volume (CTV), and adequate sparing of the sensitive tissues, a computer floppy disk is made that will be utilized to execute the delivery of the plan, during the actual treatment of the patient.

IMRT TREATMENT DELIVERY

IMRT treatment delivery is accomplished by utilizing a number of technical approaches, including static IMRT delivered with the aid of MLC, dynamic IMRT delivered with the aid of MLC and rotational tomotherapy IMRT delivered with a MIMiC (MULTIVANE INTENSITY MODULATION COMPENSATOR). Each of these techniques require the same step wise image acquisition and planning process and is likely to have similar outcomes of treatment. However, it is the Nomos-Peacock System utilizing the MIMiC that has the largest clinical experience. In addition, it is also the technology utilized by the author of this chapter, so the explanation of the IMRT treatment delivery will focus on the use of this system.

The Nomos-Peacock System utilizes a treatment method called tomotherapy, in which treatments are delivered in a series of segments or steps, through the target volume, in a rotational fashion. As the linear accelerator gantry rotates around the patient's target volume, the MIMiC under computer control, modulates the radiation beam in accordance with the dose intensity map developed by the treatment planning computer. The MIMiC can treat each segment in .5 cm, 1 cm, or 2 cm slices. The MIMiC treats two slices at a time, so that the target may be treated in 1 cm, 2 cm, or 4 cm slices thicknesses with each step. If the target is larger, or irregularly shaped the treatment table is indexed or stepped between 1 and 6 times, so as to achieve coverage of the prostate target. It is common to utilize between 2 and 3 steps for the treatment of prostate cancer. The indexing or stepping is accomplished by a device called a CRANE, which precisely moves the treatment table between each step. The MIMiC produces beam modification by dividing the collimated larger broad beamed radiation into 40 beamlets using 40 tungsten leaves, each 1 cm wide, 8 cm deep, which moves in and out of the beam's path at extremely high speeds, as the linear accelerator gantry rotates around the patient. This dynamic process allows the intensity of the beam, to vary from zero to 100% for each 5 degrees of rotation of the linear accelerator gantry. While the MIMiC's leaves move extremely rapidly to allow for the dynamic treatment process, other treatment systems utilizing conventional MLC's move much more slowly, thus requiring the use of fixed field treatment techniques, sometimes called "step and shoot".

THE FINER ASPECTS OF IMRT TREATMENT DELIVERY

The more precise one can make the dose distribution, the more precise the treatment set up must be to prevent missing the treatment target. An immobilization device, which is custom molded to each individual patient's pelvis, torso and thighs is fabricated to ensure limitation of the external motion of the patient. In addition, reproducible placement of the patient's hands and feet are also felt to be critical factors limiting external movement of the patient.

Internal movement of the prostate is a well documented phenomena, which was previously noted in the external beam radiation therapy literature, as well as observed by those radiation oncologist with extensive experience in interstitial implant techniques, which visualize the prostate in real time, under fluoroscopic and ultrasound control. Methods of internal immobilization of the prostate remain controversial, but include simple use of external immobilization devices only, bladder filling or emptying, rectal balloon to compress the prostate, new ultrasound field placement devices and the use of certain on-line portal imaging devices. At this time, it is unclear which, if any of these modalities is superior in achieving the goal of internal immobilization of the prostate.

RESULTS OF TREATMENT WITH IMRT

Long term data of treatment related side effects and efficacy are simply not available at this time. What we do know now is very encouraging. Well over 1,000 patients have been treated with IMRT for prostate cancer. Most radiation oncologists and medical physicist agree, that this technology can deliver the intended dose of radiation to the prostate, while minimizing the dose to the bladder and rectum. In fact, a paper presented at the American Association of Physicists and Medicine in 1999, showed that IMRT when compared to 3D CRT delivered 7% higher dose to the prostate, while a 9% lower dose to the bladder and a 12% lower dose to the rectum.

Moreover, several investigators report less gastrointestinal and genitourinary accute toxicity associated with IMRT, when compared with 3D CRT. Butler published a paper noting that 52% of IMRT patients had no genitourinary toxicity related to treatment, while 56.7% of patients treated with 3D CRT suffered grade 1 toxicity in a series published by Pollack. In the same group of patients 74% were treated with IMRT experienced no gastrointestinal related acute toxicity, while 66.7% experienced grade 2 acute toxicity, which required medication to control diarrhea with 3D CRT. This information is not derived from randomized data, but does suggest substantially fewer treatment related symptoms in patients receiving IMRT versus patients receiving 3D CRT.

DOSE SPECIFICATION WITH IMRT

Currently no standard convention exists to specify dose when utilizing IMRT. The nominal daily dose and total prescribed treatment dose are felt to be somewhat lower than the actual dose the prostate receives. Also, it should be noted that there is dose inhomogeneity with minimum dose regions as well as maximum dose regions similar to what is seen with interstitial implant dosimetry. Due to this fact, one should be cautious when comparing treatment doses given with IMRT to 3D CRT. Analysis of IMRT dosimetry, utilizing mean average dose methodology, for example, shows that IMRT treatment delivers significantly higher dose to the prostate when compared to conventional treatment, even though the same daily prescribed dose is administered. For example, in one model 7,000 centigray prescribed in 35 fractions, with IMRT was equivalent to the dose escalated total of approximately 7,500 centigray, when mean dose methodology was used to determine the prescribed dose. A strategy which takes advantage of this increased daily dose to the prostate, which incidentally is noted to be well tolerated, can decrease the time in which treatment is given. Kuplian has reported this modification of a treatment approach, which is sometimes called accelerated fractionation, which allowed dose escalation treatment to be delivered over less time, but with no greater side effects or morbidity. This approach may have biological advantage in terms of killing cancer cells, as well as economic advantage of shortening the treatment time.

THE PROMISE OF IMRT

The current status with regards to the evaluation of the efficacy and the effectiveness of IMRT in the treatment of prostate cancer is in much the same place 3D CRT was in the mid 1990's. However, it was the patients treated with that new treatment modality then, who comprised the data, which show the benefits of 3D CRT now. IMRT, due to its inherent precision creates new technological challenges, which are being studied and evaluated. The technology of IMRT with its precision of treatment delivery, is particularly suited to the treatment of prostate cancer and it is the view of the author, that it will fast become the technological standard to compare other external beam techniques. Does that mean the end of 3D conformal therapy, or even the replacement of many of the interstitial implants used in the treatment of prostate cancer? IMRT like the other treatment methods will find its niche and will be applied to appropriate clinical situations. The IMRT has clear advantages in terms of its precise delivery of radiation to eradicate cancer. IMRT will move from being "THE NEW - NEW THING", to an accepted and possibly superior treatment modality and its use will elevate the standard of care in the future.

Chapter 12

CYROSURGERY OF THE PROSTATE

Stuart Fisher, MD
Assistant Professor of Urology
UCLA School of Medicine
Past President
Society of Urological Cryosurgeons

HISTORY

One of the newer methods of treating localized prostate cancer is by freezing. If cells are subjected to very low temperatures, they die. The temperature needed to cause cell death ranges between -20 and -40 degree Centigrade. That's approximately minus 100 degrees Fahrenheit. Cells die because of two causes: The first is the mechanical shearing of their delicate membranes and internal anatomy by the forces of intracellular ice and the second is by changing the concentration of their intracellular fluid. When frozen, water is taken out of solution and the cells become very concentrated. With thawing, water rushes back into the cells and they pop or hemolize. Simply put, if one can lower the temperature of a cell to an extremely low temperature, the cell dies.

Freezing has been used therapeutically by dermatologists and gynecologists for many years. Warts, keratoses, seeds and superficial basal cell cancers die with the application of topical liquid nitrogen. Similarly, the application of liquid nitrogen to the cervix will cause chronically inflamed tissue to die, and slough, and be replaced by healthy new tissue. This precedence for the use of freezing therapeutically began long ago.

In the 1960's, urologists at various centers were intrigued with the possible use of freezing to treat prostate cancer. Trials were begun and a technique was established. The prostate gland was surgically exposed either through the perineum or the abdomen and a large probe was applied to the outside of the prostate gland. Liquid nitrogen was sent through the probe and an ice ball of frozen prostate gland was formed. The urologist would determine adequacy of freezing by both observing the ice ball and by feeling the prostate gland. Once it seemed that the entire gland was frozen, the probe was removed and the incision closed. The results were disastrous. Nearly every patient developed complications. There were fistulas (abnormal communications) from the prostate to the skin or from the prostate to the rectum. There were strictures (narrowing) within the prostate which did not allow urine to pass. There were strictures in the urethra. In all, it was an entirely unsuccessful venture and was abandoned.

In the 1980's transrectal ultrasonography became popular and widely accepted. The prostate is only 3 or 4 millimeters from the rectal wall and is located very close to the anal opening. This new technology provided an opportunity for better and easier view and study of the prostate. Transrectal utrasonography allowed the examiner the ability to see the entire prostate and adjacent organs. In no time, it became the standard technique used to biopsy the prostate. Previously, biopsies were done blindly by passing needles alongside a finger in the rectum. Now, one could actually see where the biopsies were being taken and even direct the biopsy needle into suspicious areas. It was a milestone.

In 1990, Onlik and Cohen, at Allegheny General Hospital in Pittsburg, began a clever project. Utilizing transrectal prostate ultrasound, they were able to guide a cryoprobe into the prostate through the perineum and freeze the prostate. They were able to monitor the freeze with ultrasound and prevented injury to the urethra and bladder by positioning a warming urethral catheter. They used liquid nitrogen and eventually utilized a series of cryoprobes to adequately freeze the entire prostate gland. With skill and experience, this technique could be performed in a minimally invasive manner with little or no bleeding or pain. The results were very good and the complications rare. It was an entirely new way of treating localized prostate cancer.

By 1994, there were more than 100 centers throughout the country performing prostate cryosurgery. Results and complications varied with skill and experience. As the procedure became more widespread there was a growing concern that it was being overdone and over promoted. In an attempt to slow down it's progress, the urethral warming catheter was recalled by the Food and Drug Administration and there was a sudden steep rise in complications. Soon the procedure was abandoned since there was no way to avoid the complications of stricture without adequate warming. After a year, the Food and Drug Administration approved the warming catheter usage and cryosurgery resumed. By 1999, Medicare approved the procedure as one of the methods of treating prostate cancer and by 2000 they included rcimbursement for patients having cryosurgery in the face of radiation therapy failure.

In 2000, many centers began using cryoprobes to treat kidney cancers both with open surgical and laparoscopic techniques. Oncologic surgeons continue to get good results by freezing liver tumors, liver metastases and bone tumors. With time, there are more and more applications of this technique to tumor treatment.

TECHNIQUE OF PROSTRATE CRYOSURGERY

The patient is given either a spinal or general anesthetic and placed in lithomy position (lying on his back with his legs apart). Cystoscopy is performed and a small tube is placed through the lower abdomen into the bladder. This a suprapupbic tub and it will be left in place to drain the bladder after the cryosurgery since the prostate will often swell after being frozen. Next the urethral warming catheter will be placed to preserve the urethra, urinary sphincter and bladder neck from being injured during the freeze. Thermocouples will be placed at strategic areas to monitor the temperature so that the surgeon can be assured that the temperature is adequately low enough to kill the tissue and that the adjacent vital structures have not been harmed. The technique is to begin the freeze anteriorly (the front portion of the prostate nearest the bladder) and to continue the freeze posteriorly (toward the back of the prostate all the way to the tip of apex). By regulating the various cryoprobes, this can be done with safety and success. After the initial freeze, the cryoprobes may be pulled back to treat any of the tissue not covered or they can be left in place for a second freeze-thaw cycle. The time needed for this technique is between 1.5 and 3 hours. After finishing the freeze, the small puncture wounds where the cryoprobes were inserted are each closed with a single absorbable stitch. The urethral warming catheter is then replaced with a conventional urethral catheter and saline is run through the suprapubic tube and out the urethral catheter so that no clots form in the bladder. The patient is then sent to a recovery room until awake and alert, and from there to his hospital room where he will be able to eat and drink. The following morning the urethral catheter is removed and the suprapubic tube is connected to a drainage bag. The patient is then discharged to return home. The blood loss for this procedure is minimal (usually less than 100 cc's) and the patients rarely require pain medication. By 4 or 5 days after the procedure, most patients are voiding satisfactorily and the suprapubic tube can be removed painlessly in the physician's office. Within a week, the majority of patients have resumed all of their usual physical activities.

WHAT TO EXPECT

With a resumption of voiding, many patients will notice urgency and an inability to hold their urine as long as they could be before the procedure. This is common and improves over a few weeks. There is also some pink tinged drainage from the urethra and occasionally a small clot might pass. The area where the cryoprobes were placed will heal very rapidly and typically the stitches will be absorbed within one or two weeks. As time passes, urinary frequency will subside and there will be marked improvement in the urinary stream. All the patients will develop erectile dysfunction. Since the nerves for potency have been frozen, there will be no spontaneous erections until the nerves regenerate. This may take between 12 to 18 months years. In the interim, the patient will need to use pills or injectables to have an erection. The ejaculation will be dry.

Three months after the procedure, a PSA will be drawn and the results will be of great importance. If the PSA is undetectable, <0 2ng/ml, the prognosis is excellent. If there is a PSA of >0.2ng/ml, there is either residual local cancer or perhaps metastatic cancer. The monthly rate of rise of the PSA can often differentiate local from metastatic disease since metastatic cancer has a very high rate of ascent.

If the PSA rises slowly but consecutively over a three month period, the prostate gland should be rebiopsied to rule out residual cancer. If present, the treatment options include repeat Cryosurgery, radiation therapy, radical surgery or hormonal ablation. All treatment options are still available.

RESULTS

If one elects to treat the prostate cancer and leave the prostate in the body, this is an in situ treatment. To date, only radiation therapy and cryosurgery are approved by Medicare for this approach. An analysis of the published peer review data comparing radiation therapy and cryosurgery revealed that both were safe and effective and nearly comparable.

Cryosurgery is minimally invasive, well tolerated, not particularly painful or debilitating and very technologically dependable. The side effects, risks and hazards are similar to the other treatment choices although some radiation therapy side effects such as radiation cystitis or proctitis may occur years after treatment, unlike surgery or cryosurgery.

Cryosurgery is the only modality which can be repeated on the same patient if the first treatment was unsuccessful.

With present techniques, cryosurgery can yield an undetectable PSA in approximately 85% of patients and carries an overall complication rate of approximately 10%. Since it is a newer treatment, there is not long term data. But then, long term data on radiation therapy and radical surgery have not been outstanding.

WHO SHOULD HAVE CRYOSURGERY?

Patients must have localized prostate cancer with no evidence of spread outside the prostate. If the PSA is higher than 10 ng/ml they should have a bone scan and CT scan to rule out metastases. There is no age distinction, but there are some qualifications. If the patient is in his 50's or 60's, he should definitely tend toward surgery since his life expectancy is 20+ years. If a patient is in his 80's, even minimally invasive surgery carries increased risks and perhaps one should consider hormonal ablation. Patients with inflammatory bowel disease such as ileitis or ulcerative colitis should not have radiation therapy and would be suitable for cryosurgery. Patients with debilitating illness requiring anticoagulation must have consent of their primary physician to discontinue anticoagulation for at least one week if they select cryosurgery. The size of the prostate gland is critically important. If the volume of the gland is greater than 40 gms (walnut size) the prostate will need to be reduced with androgen ablation prior to treatment. The smaller volume the gland, the easier to freeze. Patients concerned about potency should recognize that freezing will result in impotency and that while there is a good chance the nerves will regenerate in a year, there is no guarantee. Alternative measures such as medicine or injectables will provide a suitable erection. Patients who have had previous radiation therapy and have local recurrence are often suitable for cryosurgery. Medicare now reimburses this procedure for patients who have localized recurrence with a PSA of 8 or less and a Gleason Score of 8 or less. The usual patient for cryosurgery is a man in his 60's to 70's with a PSA of 10 or less and a Gleason Score of 6. He selects this type of treatment because he is either unable or unwilling to have radical surgery or radiation therapy.

Perhaps he has had prior radiation therapy which failed locally. Often he wants to stop hormonal therapy because of the side effects. He has learned of Cryosurgery through the Internet or media and is anxious to try something new. At present there are about 30 centers in the United States offering this therapy.

Chapter 13

EARLY HORMONE BLOCKADE IN MEN SUITABLE FOR LOCAL THERAPY

Dr. Mark Scholz & Dr. Richard Lam

Hormone blockade has historically been reserved for treatment of the advanced stages of prostate cancer, after it has metastasized to bone. In the past five years, however, several studies that were started in the early 1990s have matured, and these studies have confirmed that earlier administration of hormone blockade dramatically increases its effectiveness, prolonging life and reducing prostate cancer mortality. These recent articles have engendered a dramatic increase in the use of Early Hormone Blockade (EHB).

This chapter focuses on when and how to use EHB for newly diagnosed men who would be candidates for local therapy with surgery or radiation. Men who are diagnosed with disease too advanced for local therapy are almost always candidates for hormone blockade. However, they have additional medical needs beyond the scope of this chapter.

WHAT ARE THE CONTROVERSIES ABOUT EARLY HORMONE BLOCKADE?

Soon after prostate cancer is diagnosed, patients are confronted with an array of treatment decisions. Frequently, treatment decisions are delegated to the patients themselves, yet physicians often provide only limited guidance as to the likely outcomes of these various options. We believe it is very helpful for patients to understand some of the reasons for all the controversy.

Prostate cancer that can be detected only by abnormal elevation of PSA can almost be considered a brand new disease. Although PSA screening first became commercially available in 1988, the power and accuracy of the test were not widely recognized until the early 1990s. PSA-detected prostate cancer differs from what most physicians have historically learned about prostate cancer in medical school. In the past, physicians frequently heard the wishful statement, "If only they had caught it sooner." Now, with early diagnosis by PSA, most patients are diagnosed at the "sooner" stage. It is true that diagnosing the disease this early creates new treatment dilemmas because of the variety of potentially curative approaches and the possibility of overly aggressive treatment. However, since the tumor is likely to be much smaller than physicians traditionally have had to deal with, early PSA diagnosis unquestionably improves prostate cancer outcomes. Moreover, physicians can now track the cancer's progress after earlier treatment so they can start additional therapy earlier if the initial treatment choice does not prove to be curative.

Hormone blockade therapy is based in depriving the cancer cells of an essential growth factor, testosterone. The removal of the testosterone causes the cells to cease growing and die. Early hormone blockade, the subject of this article, is administering hormone blockade at or around the same time that local therapy is administered in an attempt to improve cure rates. (Local therapy is a general term for the different treatments done to the prostate such as Surgery, Radiation, Brachytherapy, or Cryotherapy). Typically in the past hormone blockade has only been administered after cancer had relapsed.

Not every physician believes in the effectiveness of EHB. We should not be too surprised that there is disagreement about such a new form of therapy. There are always fast and slow adopters of any new technology. Physicians, just like patients, have been slow to accept that medicines in the form of pills or shots can actually kill cancer cells! Cancer's deadliness and irreversibility have been famous for millennia. Previously the only hopes were to cut it out or burn it out.

Physicians even more than patients struggle to believe in these new treatment approaches. In the case of EHB, physicians treating prostate cancer are already very familiar with the use of hormone blockade medicines for treating advanced bone cancer. Ironically, that experience, which is not always favorable, may lead to doubts about the effectiveness of EHB. They know that the effectiveness of HB in advanced disease is usually limited to only a year or two of benefit. And this known limited benefit period in the advanced stages of disease -- the stage most physicians have treated with HB -- has no doubt created pessimism about the therapeutic potential of hormone blockade in the early-stage patients. However studies are now starting to come out showing the dramatically enhanced effectiveness of using hormone blockade right away instead of waiting. Physician's attitudes are starting to change in favor of EHB as more studies become available

What IS THE TERM "HORMONE BLOCKADE"?

When used in the context of prostate cancer, the term "Hormone Blockade" describes treatment reducing the activity of testosterone, the male hormone. Testosterone is a hormone secreted into the blood by the testicles (and to some degree the adrenal glands). Testosterone causes secondary male characteristics such as muscle and hair growth, increased libido, and the enlargement of sexual glands and organs. The prostate exists in a vestigial state before puberty and will not develop without a large increase in testosterone blood levels that occur at puberty. Therefore, the cells that make up the prostate gland are inordinately sensitive to the presence or absence of testosterone in the blood. This sensitivity can be exploited advantageously as a therapy for prostate cancer because prostate cancer cells are derived from the prostate gland and retain the need for testosterone to remain viable. This need for testosterone is unique to prostate cancer and is almost universally present when prostate cancer is still in its early stages.

Hormone blockade. deprives prostate cancer cells of testosterone. When deprived of testosterone, the cancer cells actually commit suicide in a cell death process called apoptosis. The prostate cancer cell, because it retains the lineage of a normal prostate gland cell, responds to the hormonal signal of low testosterone blood levels by releasing enzymes internally that cause self-destruction. The amount of cell death in early-stage prostate cancer is usually dramatic. On rare occasions, no cancer at all can be found in men undergoing surgery after HB. More typically, there is a dramatic reduction in the number of cancer cells, but not total elimination. In some cases, particularly in men with higher grade cancer or more locally advanced disease, the HB effect is limited to minor shrinkage.

Hormone blockade also appears to have the ability to put some prostate cancer cells to "sleep." What all this means is that the effect of HB on different cells in a prostate cancer tumor can be variable. Many of the cancer cells are killed, but others are simply inhibited from growing. Why some cells are killed and others only inhibited is an active area of prostate cancer research.

The commonly used medicines that accomplish hormone blockade in patients with early disease fall into two categories: In the first category are the LHRH agonists Lupron or Zoladex, medicines that stop testosterone production in the testicles. They are administered by intramuscular injection every 1-4 months. In the other category of medication are those that block testosterone from activating the prostate cancer cell directly. These agents, Casodex or Flutamide, are administered in pill form on a once or twice daily basis.

These two classes of therapeutic agents can be used either by themselves or in combination in an attempt to attain a more powerful therapeutic effect. The advantages and disadvantages of using agents singly or in combination in early stage disease have not been determined since no studies yet exist directly addressing this question in early stage disease. Most high quality studies published to date have used a single agent from the first category(LHRH agonists). In our medical practice at this time, it is our policy to use one agent from the first category (Lupron or Zoladex) in combination with an agent from the second category (Casodex or Flutamide). Usually the Casodex or Flutamide pills are started a week prior to the first shot of Lupron or Zoladex to block the initial testosterone flare the shots induce.

WHAT ARE THE GOALS OF EARLY HORMONE BLOCKADE ?

1) Improving Survival

The most common motivation for adding EHB to radiation or surgery is to improve the cure rate and reduce the chance that the cancer will relapse in the future. Some studies evaluating hormone blockade added to radiation use relatively short courses of HB lasting three to eight months. One study of HB added to radiation directly compared three months of HB with eight months of HB. The study concluded that the patients treated with eight months of HB had a significant reduction in their risk of relapse, but no improvement in survival, compared to the patients who had only three months of HB. In this study the patients were started on the radiation and HB at the same time. The hormone blockade was continued after the radiation was completed.

Another important study of HB added to radiation compared the use of HB for a total of three years to the use of hormone blockade added when and if the patient relapsed. This study was done with 400 patients who had large cancers that could be felt digitally in the prostate or who had high Gleason scores. Patient evaluation for study purposes occurred five years after starting the radiation. In the group of two hundred patients who only had HB therapy when and if they relapsed, 26 died of prostate cancer within that five-year period. In the other group of 200 men, who had EHB with their radiation, only six died of prostate cancer within five years. Moreover, 85% percent of the men who had EHB were without evidence of cancer after five years. On the other hand, only 48% of the 200 men who had delayed HB were free of cancer by that time. One cannot help but wonder if the same beneficial effect of EHB can be accomplished with a shorter period of HB. In fact, a similar study demonstrated a beneficial effect of EHB after 28 months of therapy.

Another recent study looked at hormone blockade added to surgery in 100 volunteers whose prostate cancer was found to have spread to their lymph nodes at the time of radical Prostatectomy. Forty-eight men were randomly selected to receive EHB within 12 weeks of having the surgery, and the HB was continued indefinitely. The other 52 men started HB treatment only if they had disease recurrence and evidence of clinical progression. This means that the men who had the delayed HB were not generally treated if they simply had a rising PSA without symptoms related to prostate cancer.

Seven years after the surgery, the 48 men treated with EHB manifested a seven-fold reduction in prostate cancer mortality: only two of them had died of prostate cancer. Unfortunately, 17 out of the 52 men treated with delayed HB had died of prostate cancer. Moreover, 38 of the 48 EHB patients were free of evidence of prostate cancer including PSA evidence. On the other hand, only seven of the surviving men who were treated with delayed HB were free of evidence of active cancer.

These high-quality randomized prospective studies conclusively show the advantages of using EHB, especially in men with higher grade or more locally advanced disease. One important unanswered question is whether or not such long treatment periods are necessary to obtain these favorable results. Clearly, studies show that eight months of HB is suboptimal. Twenty-eight months appears to be the minimum treatment period that should be considered if patients and physicians are using HB to increase the cure rate of local therapy. It is possible that eighteen months will be beneficial, but we do not have enough data to currently draw that conclusion.

However, longer treatment periods come at the cost of increased side effects from HB. Hormone blockade administered for more than two years engenders a rising risk of permanent testosterone loss especially in men over age 70. There is also some evidence that a proportion of men treated with hormone blockade will not recover normal sexual desire even if their male hormone levels do recover. Most other side effects are reversible or treatable. This issue is addressed somewhat further below. At the time of writing this chapter, our policy (when the goal of HB is reduction in relapse risk) is to recommend a minimum of eight months treatment. The patients who have prostate cancer with higher-grade elements are considered for longer treatment periods of 12-18 months unless side effects from HB become excessive. Patients whose cancer has spread to the lymph nodes or who show other signs of a commensurate stage disease probably should consider doing a full three years of EHB.

2) Reducing Side Effects of Radiation

Hormone blockade administered to patients with early-stage prostate cancer can be implemented for purposes other than increasing the cure rate of radiation or surgery. Hormone blockade not only kills prostate cancer cells, it also kills prostate gland cells, causing the prostate gland to shrink. Shrinkage of the prostate gland can be advantageous before treatment with radiation, particularly seed radiation. The radiation therapist can then limit the extent of treatment to the smaller area represented by the diminished prostate. This can be an important benefit because there is a risk of urinary blockage after a seed implantation, and this risk rises with the size of the prostate gland. In fact, many reputable centers will not implant prostates that have a volume greater than 60cc (measured on ultrasound). Men who have 3-6 months of HB treatment will, on average, see a 50% reduction in prostate size. Hence, this shrinking effect of HB on the prostate gland allows some men with large prostates to more safely undergo seed implantation radiation therapy.

Shrinking the prostate with EHB prior to conformal beam radiation reduces the side effects of this type of radiation also. Large prostates often protrude into the rectal vault such that conformal radiation ends up treating a much greater amount of the rectal wall than is desirable. Shrinking the prostate down so that it does not protrude into the rectal vault minimizes the amount of radiation that is directed to the rectum and this reduces the chance of long term rectal side effects such rectal bleeding.

3) Estimating Cancer Relapse Risk

How much the PSA drops in the initial months after starting HB adds additional information about the aggressiveness of the cancer in that specific individual and helps uncover patients who are more likely to relapse in the future. One study used a PSA cut-off point of 0.5 three months after starting HB (in this study the radiation was started three months after the HB was started). Five years after radiation (and HB), 74% of the men whose PSA had dropped to less than 0.5 were still in complete remission without evidence of recurrent cancer. Conversely, only 40% of the men whose PSA was greater than 0.5 three months after starting HB were still in complete remission five years later. In other words, the PSA behavior just three months after starting HB would enable physicians to predict a greater than two-fold increase in relapse risk. The results of this study strongly suggest that radiation should not be started until the behavior of the PSA under the influence of HB has been determined. Men whose PSA does not drop below 0.5 three months after starting HB should carefully consider continuing their HB for at least eight months if not substantially longer.

Who Are Candidates for Primary HB Therapy?

Hormone blockade is the only form of prostate cancer therapy that has been proven to prolong life in randomized prospective trials. (Randomized prospective trials for surgery and radiation cannot be done because of the natural unwillingness of patients to have their treatment assigned randomly.) Randomized trials comparing hormone blockade alone with hormone blockade plus radiation are presently in process. The question being asked in these trials is whether or not the radiation is contributing anything of importance to survival above what the HB is already accomplishing.

We and others have been using HB as sole therapy in early-stage patients for as long as 10 years. Hormone blockade is administered either continuously or intermittently. The development of hormone resistance within five years of starting treatment appears to be a very rare event as long as there is a good initial decline in PSA after starting HB. We like to see the PSA below 0.2 after three months and less than 0.05 after six months of HB. Patients with early-stage disease who achieve this type of PSA response clearly have hormone-sensitive disease that has a very high likelihood of remaining so for many years.

Since hormone resistance is a rare phenomenon in this group of patients, we have taken to stopping HB after 12-16 months in an attempt to reduce the side effects of HB and improve the patient's quality of life. We find that after HB is stopped, it takes an average of five months for the testosterone to recover to the normal range. Patients are then able to stay off treatment for an average of 18 months before the PSA rises back up to an arbitrary level of 5.0. Proscar administered in a dose of 5mg per day during the time after the HB is stopped can further slow the rate of PSA rise. On average, it adds an additional year of "off time" to that otherwise anticipated. Hormone resistance in a population of early-stage patients defined by a good initial PSA decline is practically nonexistent within the first five years after starting HB. One sees the evidence of this persistent hormone sensitivity when restarting HB. The PSA drop in response to starting the HB for the second cycle, mirrors the decline seen when HB was initially started.

In summary, Early Hormone Blockade has several potential benefits. The most notable benefit is its proven ability to reduce prostate cancer mortality in patients who have high-risk disease. Also, early hormone blockade can be of value in reducing side effects from radiation in patients with enlarged prostates, and measurement of the PSA three months after starting HB identifies patients at higher risk for prostate cancer relapse after radiation. Lastly, EHB can be a first step for patients who are undecided about what form of local therapy to choose, and EHB may be an option for patients who want to forgo local therapy altogether. The early response to HB as well as the individual's subjective perception of the side effects of HB allow a first hand judgment to be made as to how palatable primary HB is for him personally. If he perceives the side effects of primary HB to be too unpleasant, he can opt for local therapy with surgery or radiation at an institution of excellence.

WHEN IS EHB UNNECESSARY?

Hormone blockade is not free of side effects. However, many of the side effects such as hot flashes, weight gain, decreased muscle, fatigue, and even impotence can be ameliorated or reversed with specific therapies. One common side effect of HB that can be a problem is loss of libido. There is no effective therapy to stimulate sexual desire. The loss of interest in sex occurs in more than 90% of men treated with HB (impotence is the loss of ability to get an erection while loss of libido is defined as a lack of interest in sex or sexual desire). Of even greater concern, libido sometimes does not fully return after the HB is stopped. This problem seems to be more common in elderly men but it has also been encountered in younger men.

Therefore, situations where HB can be safely avoided need to be defined. Patients who have very high cure rates with surgery or radiation alone will experience such a small benefit from HB that the potential risk of side effects from HB outweighs the potential benefit. Take for example patients with the following characteristics:

PSA less than 10
Gleason less than 7

Clinical stage less than T2b
Number of core biopsies positive less than 33%

Individuals with cancers that meet all the above criteria have cure rates of approximately 90% ten years after local therapy (with seed implants, surgery, or conformal radiation) as long as the treatment was administered at a center of excellence. Thus, individuals who meet all the above criteria only have a 10% risk of relapse. We estimate that adding 28 months (but possibly only 18) of HB reduces the relapse rate by 50% so it will cut that 10% risk in half to 5%. In other words, the risk of relapse will go from one out of ten to one out of 20. Many men elect to forego the inconvenience and risk of side effects from EHB when the actual potential benefit is so small.

Another group of patients who might elect to forego EHB are men over age 70 who are at a somewhat higher risk of relapse than the above group of men. A "somewhat higher risk" can be defined as having all the above favorable risk factors minus one. For example:

The PSA is 10 – 20 or
The Gleason score is 7 or
The clinical stage is T2b or
The % positive biopsy cores are from 33 – 50%

Individuals who have only one of the above unfavorable factors have about a 25% chance for relapse from local therapy within 10 years. In this case, EHB treatment for18 to 28 months would reduce the chance for relapse from one in four down to one out of eight. Why would a 70 year old or older man perhaps decide to assume an increased risk of relapse? Studies of HB administered at the first sign of PSA relapse appear to indicate that control of the relapsed disease can be accomplished for 10 years or longer in a high percentage of cases. Deferring HB to the first sign of relapse enables 75% of men who have intermediate-risk disease to be cured of prostate cancer without risking permanent attenuation of libido. The other 25% would be at or beyond life expectancy before control of the relapsed disease would lose effectiveness.

Chapter 14

NEW APPROACHES TO PROSTATE CANCER TREATMENT

Dr. Mark Scholz and Dr. Richard Lam

Recent statistics show a significant reduction in the number of men dying of prostate cancer each year. Even in the face of an aging population, where more people would be expected to die. Why? The recent decline in death rates cannot be attributed to a single factor but rather to a combination of factors. It appears that a variety of incremental treatment improvements are contributing to a synergistic improvement in overall outcomes.

The treatment improvements that seem to be making the biggest impact are earlier diagnosis using PSA testing, improved biopsy techniques that find the cancer with greater regularity, and perhaps most importantly, early hormone blockade. Another factor may be that physicians are more aggressive in treating early stage disease with surgery or radiation because improved technology makes treatment less debilitating.

We're making progress through combinations of incremental improvements that together are adding up to substantially improved overall outcomes. Today, 80 to 90 percent of men diagnosed with prostate cancer will not die from it; either they will be cured by treatment or die of other causes before the cancer progresses. Therefore the development of new treatment approaches should focus on three main areas:

Development of methods, for newly diagnosed patients, to more accurately separate the minority destined to die of the disease from the majority who won't. This will allow us to intervene early with more aggressive treatment leading to higher cure rates and reduce the intensity of treatment (and side-effects) in those who have less dangerous disease.

Reduction of the side effects of existing therapies. If prostate cancer patients are going to survive, we should be developing treatments that don't devastate urinary and sexual function.

Development of new medicines and treatments to forestall death in men with metastatic disease.

1. MODERN STAGING TECHNIQUES

Presently, the first point is being addressed through the ongoing refinement of staging. A brief explanation of staging might be helpful here, since this is a rapidly evolving area.

Prostate cancer begins as a single malignant cell that grows progressively into ever-larger numbers. If allowed to proceed it eventually mutates into even more virulent clones that break free from the mother tumor and spread to form new tumors in other areas of the body usually the bone marrow or lymph nodes. Staging, for newly diagnosed prostate cancer patients, tries to help answer the important question: "Has the disease spread outside the prostate?" In its early stages of spread, when there are only a few microscopic cells outside the prostate (micro-metastatic disease), we lack adequate technology to determine exactly where the disease is located in the body. We can however predict the likelihood of such spread by looking at blood tests, scans, and biopsy results. The early stages of prostate cancer are subdivided and defined by how high the risk is for having microscopic spread of the disease outside the prostate gland. Early stage prostate cancer, disease with a reasonably good chance of being located in the prostate gland or immediate area, is divided into the three categories: Good-risk, Intermediate-risk, and High- risk.

Good-risk and Intermediate-risk prostate cancer were defined in the previous chapter.

High-risk patients have one or more of the factors listed below. They also have clear bone scans and CT scans. Their serum Prostatic Acid Phosphatase (PAP, a blood test) is normal. They have a chance for cure* with local therapy but the chance for cure is small: The percent risk of relapse for high-risk patients after radiation or surgery alone will vary from 50% to 90%. High-risk patients have at least one of the following characteristics:

High Risk Patients
- Gleason score greater than 7
- Clinical Stage of C (stage T3)
- PSA greater than 20
- Two or more of the intermediate-risk factors present

Endorectal MRI or Color Doppler Ultrasound showing penetration of the cancer outside the capsule of the prostate gland
- PSA greater than 0.5 after 3 months of Hormone Blockade

Today, most newly diagnosed patients are categorized early stage, as defined by the three risk categories above (Low, Intermediate, and High). Newly diagnosed patients can also present at a later stage, a circumstance that needs definition as well. If certain scans, blood tests, or surgical findings confirm the spread of disease beyond the area of the prostate gland, attempting to define the risk of spread becomes

---

* Patients occasionally express surprise when use the work cure while talking about prostate cancer. In the past, before the development of PSA, a serious question was raised about whether prostate cancer was ever cured. One theory was that maybe prostate cancer has always spread by the time it is diagnosed. In the era prior to PSA some men experienced years free of disease after surgery but others would have sudden relapses in the bones. So some physicians speculated that no one was ever cured. The only reason some men seemed free of disease was because in some individuals the disease was very slow growing. These physicians believed that given enough time all men would relapse.

unimportant. The Gleason score, digital rectal exam, and PSA findings are less important in these more advanced stages since the disease is already known to have spread. Below is a listing of the disease stages where there is confirmed spread of cancer:

Stage DO Patients: Serum prostatic acid phosphatase consistently elevated above the normal range with repeat testing. Bone scan and CT scan are clear

Stage D1 Patients: Confirmed spread to the lymph nodes but with a clear bone scan.

Stage D2 (Bone Scan Positive) Patients: Spread to the bones visualized on bone scan confirmed by a characteristic pattern or via other means such as x-ray or MRI

For completeness of our review of staging we should mention the last category of prostate cancer patients, those who have undergone therapy but the therapy has ceased to be effective.

PSA Relapse Patients: Relapsed after local therapy with a rising PSA who have a clear bone scan and CT scan**.

Hormone Resistant Patients: Patients with a rising PSA even though their testosterone levels are low.

2. DEFFERED THERAPY IN NEWLY-DIAGNOSED GOOD-RISK PATIENTS

The most extreme way of reducing treatment side effects is to withhold treatment altogether. Watching cancer without treatment is

---

** It is true that a minority of patients with rising PSA after local therapy will still have disease confined to the prostate or prostate area. The process of deciding whether or not to pursue further treatment to the prostate area in PSA relapse patients is an important issue too extensive to address in this chapter.

certainly an unexpected concept. Deferred therapy, called watchful waiting, has been the standard approach in the very elderly or very ill from other medical problems. This approach has also been studied in younger men in Europe. The studies show that in some patients the cancer does not progress even after 10 years.

Why would young men opt to simply watch what is a potentially curable disease? There are several answers. First it's well known that some men have a form of low-grade disease that will remain stable for many years without treatment. Presently the only way to find these non-progressing patients is by monitoring them over time. Another part of the appeal of watchful waiting is, we are in the midst of a technological revolution. Prostate cancer therapy has changed dramatically over the last 10 years and, we expect, that 10 years in the future prostate cancer treatment will in no way resemble what we see today. Present day state of the art surgery and radiation have dramatically improved. However patients cannot escape the reality that even, in the best hands, at least 5 – 10% of men undergoing surgery or radiation will suffer permanent long-term unpleasant side effects, apart from impotence, which occurs at an even higher incidence.

So it would seem that waiting for better, less invasive and debilitating treatment, makes sense if it is not too risky to wait. There are logical reasons to consider that deferred therapy in good risk patients might be safe. Presently with modern technology the cure rate in the good risk category is very high. Theoretically it is possible to select a sub-group of extra-good risk patients (PSA greater than 6.0, Gleason greater than 7, Clinical stage greater than T2b) for deferred therapy and implement treatment when they show progression yet while they are still in the good risk category (before the PSA rises above 9?). As an additional precaution other forms of testing are done with digital rectal exams, endorectal MRI scans, Color Doppler Ultrasound, or even repeat biopsies.

In my opinion, men who choose watchful waiting, should obtain a quality baseline endorectal MRI or Color Doppler Ultrasound for two reasons. First it establishes a baseline for future comparison and can be repeated annually as an independent method, apart from PSA, to monitor for any evidence of growth of the cancer. In a few years, spectroscopic enhancement of the endorectal MRI should make this form of monitoring even more useful. Second, is to detect the small percentage of good-risk patients who have more advanced disease, than a low PSA and other favorable factors would seem to indicate. Patients who are found, on endorectal MRI, to have either a large tumor or capsular penetration should be advised to forgo watchful waiting and proceed on to some form of therapy.

3. NEW DRUGS FOR ADVANCED STAGES OF PROSTATE CANCER

TAXOTERE

Chemotherapy right after surgery has become the standard approach for reducing relapse rates in breast and colon cancer. Patients with stage D1 prostate cancer have approximately a one to four or one to five chance of dying of prostate cancer within 10 to 15 years of being diagnosed, even if they have local therapy and start early hormone blockade and continue it for years. The reason is the occasional failure of local therapy and long-term hormone blockade to eradicate or at least control every single cancer cell. What happens is a small but resistant population of cells survives and over time grows to bigger and bigger proportions. Eventually the progressive disease is detected by a rising PSA and later by positive bone scans.

Adjuvant chemotherapy is the administration of chemotherapy treatment at a point when only a few resistant cells are present. The idea is to eradicate the residual clone of resistant disease when it is at an earlier, more vulnerable stage. Until recently there were no active chemotherapy agents for prostate cancer to consider for use in the adjuvant setting. Fortunately now an active form of chemotherapy called Taxotere is available. Studies using Taxotere in advanced prostate cancer show it to be two or three times more effective than other available agents. Taxotere is not yet FDA approved for prostate cancer but off label use of FDA approved drugs is a very common practice in the USA especially in the field of oncology. Any oncologist in the USA can prescribe and administer Taxotere to any patient who he feels has a realistic chance of benefiting from the therapy. The appropriate scheduling, timing, and duration of adjuvant chemotherapy have already been carefully worked out by researchers in the field of breast cancer; injections administered 3 times per month for 4 to 6 months appear to give optimal results. The side effects of Taxotere are typical of most chemotherapy and usually consists of tiredness and temporary hair loss.

CELECOXIB

Celecoxib (Celebrex) is a promising anti-cancer medication which belongs in the cox-2 inhibitor class of anti-inflammatory drugs. Celecoxib is FDA-approved for the treatment of osteoarthritis. It is thought to exert anti-cancer effect is via angiogenesis inhibition, promotion of apoptosis (programmed cell death), and decreased tumor invasiveness.

Currently, the drug is in advanced studies for colon, lung and prostate cancer. A small pilot study demonstrated that celecoxib exerted a significant effect on PSA levels in patients with biochemical progression after prostatectomy or radiation. In our experience, celecoxib is a low-toxicity drug that can often delay the need for more aggressive and potent therapy such as systemic hormone blockade.

NILUTAMIDE

Nilutamide (Nilandrone), like biclutamide and flutamide, belongs in the anti-androgen class of drugs. Its mechanism of action is via blocking testosterone from reaching the prostate cancer cell. Used in conjunction with chemical castration or orchiectomy, anti-androgens result in a higher and more dramatic PSA response rate. In our practice, we use nilutamide when the other anti-androgens have lost its effect. In our experience as well as those reported elsewhere, the success rate for nilutamide is approximately 50%. Fortunately, the PSA reducing effects can often be quite durable.

ZOLENDRONIC ACID

Zolendronic acid (Zometa) belongs in a class of drug called bisphosphonates. Zometa was FDA-approved specifically for cancer patients who have metastatic disease to the bone. Prostate cancer has a high affinity for the skeletal system, and the skeletal complications from prostate cancer can be very severe and life-altering. Zometa has been shown to significantly delay or prevent the onset of skeletal complications associated with prostate cancer.

THALIDOMIDE

Thalidomide was originally FDA approved for the treatment of morning sickness in pregnant women. It also functions as a sleeping pill. Unfortunately it causes severe birth defects since it inhibits the normal development of blood vessels. This blood vessel growth inhibiting effect is now being successfully exploited to inhibit the growth of cancer. Most research with Thalidomide is in a disease called multiple myeloma, another cancer that spreads to the bone marrow. Studies on Thalidomide report that 30% to 50% of the patients benefit, as indicated by a decline in PSA. Despite the use of high doses of Thalidomide the side effects from the treatment were mostly limited to constipation, numbness of hands and feet, and sleepiness. The tolerability of the drug makes it an attractive agent for use in combination with other active agents. Our own experience with low-dose Thalidomide (50-100mg a day) is that it actively suppresses PSA in men who are starting with relatively low PSA levels to begin with. Thalidomide appears to be an active agent for use in men with PSA relapses or in men on intermittent hormone blockade who want to extend their time off therapy.

REZULIN

Rezulin is another oral agent which until recently was on the market for the treatment of adult onset diabetes. Unfortunately the drug caused sporadic cases of liver damage rendering it unsafe for routine use in diabetics. Dr. Kantoff, at Dana Farber, recently published a trial using the drug to treat patients with prostate cancer. Only one out of 41 patients treated had to stop because of liver problems. The liver problem reversed once the drug was stopped. Of the 41 patients treated 16 stabilized their PSA levels through out the duration of the 8-month trial indicating that this drug may have substantial activity against prostate cancer.

PURELY INVESTIGATIONAL TREATMENTS

The treatments reviewed so far in this chapter are already accessible to patients in the USA through licensed medical physicians. Below are listed a couple new treatment approaches presently under investigation that will probably become available in the next few years.

MONOCLONAL ANTIBODIES

Researchers are harnessing the immune systems of animals by injecting cancer cells into mice and harvesting the antibodies for injection into humans. New technology has been used to sanitize the mouse antibodies for safe human use. The beauty of antibody technology is that these proteins can seek out and attack the cancer wherever it is in the body while completely sparing normal body tissues. It appears that such an antibody has been developed for the treatment of prostate cancer. The antibody attaches to a protein called PSMA on the surface of prostate cancer cells. Preliminary studies in humans seem to indicate that this antibody is very specific for prostate cancer. If these studies are born out, the next step will probably be to link the PSMA antibody to a radioactive source taking the radioactivity right to the surface of the cancer cell to kill it no matter where it is in the body. This same technology has already succeeded and is commercially available for the treatment of another type of cancer called lymphoma.

EPIDERMAL GROWTH FACTOR RECEPTOR INHIBITORS

It is widely believed that the epidermal growth factor receptor (EGFR) plays a role in cancer cell proliferation. Researchers have devised many novel compounds which somehow block, inhibit, or turn-off this receptor, with promising results. Two FDA-approved drugs, Iressa and Erbitux, have been shown to prolong survival in lung and colon cancer, respectively. These 2 compounds along with another one named Tarceva are all in various stages of study for prostate cancer.

GENETIC TREATMENTS

Researchers at Memorial Sloan Kettering in New York have been working on a genetically altered virus that only attacks human cells that produce PSA. That means these viruses will not replicate in normal human cells; they only grow and replicate in prostate cancer cells and the normal prostate gland cells. So far a safe way to inject the virus into the blood stream has not been developed. However injections into the area of the prostate appear to be feasible and safe. This approach is presently under investigation for men who have previously had radiation to the prostate gland as an alternative to doing surgery. Surgery on a previously radiated prostate is very risky often resulting in urinary incontinence.

All the treatment approaches discussed in this chapter are insufficiently researched for the general medical community to have yet formed a consensus regarding their effectiveness. We do not want to leave the impression that by listing these approaches, to the exclusion of other more established treatments that I am implying these approaches are necessarily superior. Good treatment decisions depend on obtaining expert advice, being fully informed of all available options, and tailoring therapies to the unique needs of each individual patient.

Once PSA was discovered physicians realized that the only men who developed relapsed cancer in the bones were those who many years before started to have a rise in PSA. The rise in PSA is now known to invariably precede the relapse of cancer in the bones. Subsequently, armed with this new knowledge, researchers began to check PSA levels regularly after surgery or radiation to see if some patients would maintain a low PSA indefinitely (beyond 5 and 10 years). In the last 3-5 years over a score of studies have come out showing that the majority of good-risk and intermediate-risk patients remain without evidence for PSA relapse 10 years after treatment. Practically all physicians these days accept that men without PSA relapse 10 years are for all intents and purposes CURED of prostate cancer.

Chapter 15

WHAT'S WRONG WITH THE WATCHFUL WAITING POSTURE THAT IS SO POPULAR IN EUROPE?

Tom Alexander

Fortune, Sept 20, 1993 v128 n6 p86(9).

One man's tough choices on prostate cancer, by Tom Alexander

Abstract: A man diagnosed with prostate cancer received many differing and sometimes contradicting opinions on how to treat it. When he set out to learn as much as he could about the disease he found he was able consult on an even level with physicians and chart his own course of treatment.

Text:

THE ASSISTANT to the prominent urological surgeon was returning my call late one evening. "You need to get into surgery right away," he said. "If you don't, the chances are about 100% that your cancer will escape the prostate in the next one to two years. Meanwhile, I'd recommend you start taking Eulexin to put it in remission, but don't rely on that for more than a month or a month and a half."

After hanging up the phone, I didn't sleep very well again that night. I had been sleeping poorly ever since the diagnosis of prostate cancer a couple of weeks earlier had shaken me out of my customary indifference to health and dropped me into a stew of controversy. It divides medical professionals and bewilders rapidly growing numbers of men.

In men the disease is already the most common cancer, and the second leading cause of cancer death after lung cancer. An estimated 165,000 new cases will be diagnosed in the U.S. this year, nearly double the 86,000 cases found in 1985. Rather than constituting a new epidemic, however, the increase mainly reflects improved ability to find tumors. Most men over 60 probably have some form of prostate cancer but don't know it.

Chances are, my own would have gone unnoticed or been found too late for treatment were it not for those new diagnostic techniques. I had finally gone in for a physical exam—something I've tended to neglect since retiring to western North Carolina and escaping company-mandated physicals. My physician mentioned that his digital-rectal exam showed I had an enlarged prostate, which I already knew, but he suspected it to be the benign condition common in men my age, which is 62.

Still, he said, the blood test indicated a PSA level of 5.9. He explained that PSA stands for "prostate-specific antigen," which normally ranges between 1 and 4. While somewhat higher readings often merely reflect benign enlargements, they can also indicate cancer. (I knew none of this. In recent years I've tended to tune out the conversation of old cronies, dwelling as it does on things like diet, cholesterol, and PSA instead of hunting, fishing, and girls.) The physician suggested I visit a urologist, which I eventually got around to doing.

Besides PSA analysis, the urologist deployed another new technique, using an ultrasound instrument that assembles echoes from high-frequency sound waves into fuzzy images of the walnut-size prostate gland, which is just below the bladder. As the uncomfortable rectal procedure continued, he spotted a couple of suspicious regions, and ultrasonically guided a hollow needle into each to extract tiny cores of tissue.

On my next appointment, he reported that the local pathologist had found "something unusual" on one of the slides and had sent them off to a prominent pathologist they sometimes consult at Johns Hopkins Hospital in Baltimore. Mildly alarmed at last, I asked him how often this expert confirmed the presence of cancer in cases like mine. "Almost always," he said, his voice finally softening, and he leaned over and patted my knee.

The Johns Hopkins expert indeed reported cancer on one of the slides, describing it as "a moderately differentiated adenocarcinoma," with a Gleason score of 3+2. As I later learned, differentiation and Gleason grades measure the state of development of cancer cells as seen through a microscope. To the expert eye, normal prostate cells are readily identifiable and thus called highly differentiated. As cancer's out-of-control growth proceeds, cells lose this differentiation, mutating into five characteristic patterns. These patterns can be graded from 1 to 5 on the Gleason scale, the higher numbers indicating less differentiation and thus greater malignancy. A Gleason score consists of the grades of the two most prevalent cancer cell populations.

The overwhelming concern about prostate cancer is its potential for metastasis—for cells to escape the gland and take root in lymph nodes, bones, lungs, skin, or other tissue. As long as it is truly confined, it is completely curable; once it spreads it is no longer considered curable, but it can be controlled to a degree by depriving it of the hormone, testosterone, that seems to fuel its growth. Testosterone can either be removed at its source, through orchiectomy (castration), or blocked by administering female hormones or other chemicals such as Eulexin.

My next step was a bone scan at a local hospital to see whether cancer was already in the bones. Late that same afternoon I proceeded once more to the urologist's office. Since whatever lay ahead inevitably involved my wife, Jane, I suggested she come along.

The urologist opened with the welcome news that the bone scan appeared negative. He said I probably had a small, localized tumor in one lobe of the gland. A major unknown was the status of my lymph nodes, but assuming they too were negative, he went on, the primary treatment options were surgery and radiation.

Surgery meant a radical Prostatectomy, which entails removing the entire prostate plus some amount of surrounding tissue. It would have the built-in advantage that, once I was opened up, the surgeon's first act would be to have my pelvic lymph nodes examined. If they proved cancerous, the Prostatectomy would be halted and I would be stitched up and put on hormone treatments.

If I opted for radiation, he suggested that I first undergo a laparoscopic examination of the lymph nodes, which is done with a long manipulator that is inserted through small holes made in the abdomen and guided by fiber optics. Again assuming negative nodes, the radiation treatment he recommended was the external-beam variety, which entails projecting high-energy X-rays through the body, converging on the prostate.

HE EXPLAINED that the cure rate for surgery is about 95%, and for radiation, 75% to 85%. Each treatment carries its own risks. With surgery, a man my age stands a 50% to 75% chance of being rendered impotent—despite the celebrated "nerve-sparing" techniques pioneered at Johns Hopkins in the mid-1980s. With radiation, he said, the odds of becoming impotent are 20% to 40%. With either treatment, I stood about a 3% chance of becoming permanently incontinent—unable to control urine. (As I later discovered, some surveys indicate considerably higher failure rates for both treatments, and in the case of surgery, higher probabilities of complete or partial incontinence plus risks of cardiopulmonary troubles, urine blockage, and rectum or bowel injury.

Radiation, the urologist continued, posed a 2% or 3% risk of damaging the bowel, bladder, or other organs. Finally, radical

Prostatectomy carried about a 1% chance of death, but since I was a "young" man in apparent good health, he considered me an excellent surgery candidate. (Among the few compensations of my medical situation—aside from the spice it adds to retirement - is constantly being referred to as "young" in urological circles.) According to the urologist, the surgery would involve about five days in the hospital and a convalescence of six to eight weeks. Radiation would entail six weeks of five-days-a-week treatments.

At that point I asked what would happen if I simply did nothing. The physician's words clattered back like chips of ice: The probability of my cancer metastasizing during the next five years was about 40%. Once that happened, hormone treatments might keep it under control for around 2 1/2 years before further deterioration set in. Then I might expect pain, kidney obstructions, anemia, weakness, and death. At the end of the session, I asked the urologist what he would do in my shoes, and without hesitation he said he'd have a radical Prostatectomy.

Jane and I drove home through the winter night, hearts chilling. To the American mind, cancer seems the ultimate catastrophe, far more fearsome than hypertension or emphysema, which can make you just as dead. Amid bouts of depression, I began trying, as so many others have, to comprehend what life had pitched at me and what to do about it. I had spent a good deal of my career reporting on science and technology and their many controversies, but I was unfamiliar with medicine and taken aback by the rampant disarray in the field of prostate cancer, where seemingly all the experts disagreed and nothing was certain except the inexorably growing malignancy at the seat of my being.

My point of entry into the maze was the National Cancer Institute's information service hotline—800-4-CANCER—staffed by energetic and well-informed folks who calmly answer patients' and physicians' questions, dispatch the institute's numerous free publications, and call up knowledge from its databanks.

For me, the service's most useful output was the PDQ (for Physician Data Query) Treatment Information for Prostate Cancer, a constantly updated summary of state-of-the-art therapy recommendations. PDQ's extensive bibliography kept Jane busy tracking down journal articles at a local medical library, the Mountain Area Health Education Center in Asheville. The cheery hotline people also mentioned various prostate cancer patient support groups, notably Us Too—men's belated counterpart to Y-Me?, the women's breast-cancer group. Us Too has chapters all over the country where patients meet to exchange information and experiences.

One evening Jane and I attended an Us Too session and were struck by the tales recounted. One man, who appeared to be in his late 50s, said he had been diagnosed with the disease a few years earlier, shortly after marrying his attractive, younger-looking wife, who was also present. Concerned about impotence, he had elected a somewhat controversial radiation-implant procedure wherein tiny radioactive seeds are planted directly inside the prostate, the idea being to deliver heavier doses to the tumor than the external beam procedure does while reducing damage to other tissue. In this man's case, the treatment had failed to eradicate the cancer, so his PSA levels were rising again. I inquired whether he now regretted his treatment decision, and he happily replied, "Not at all. We've had several years of wonderful sex, which we might otherwise not have had."

Another man, far less content, repeatedly complained that he had been rushed into radical Prostatectomy without a full understanding of the possible outcomes. By now, he was impotent and incontinent and still had his cancer. "I wish I had taken more time," he kept saying.

In the weeks that followed, I thought a lot about those two stories. I am sexually active, as the current phrase puts it, but when I raise concerns about impotence, many urologists impatiently dismiss them, though some mention the existence of prostheses and injections to deal with the problem. Moreover, I lead a pretty active and satisfying outdoor life in the Great Smoky Mountains and recognize that any complications from treatment would probably be with me the rest of my days, while the benefits would not accrue for years, if ever.

My father, a hearty, kinetic outdoor type, was once induced by stomach pains to submit to an exploratory operation when he, like me, was in his early 60s. The surgeons never found anything and the stomach pains eventually went away, but in the decade of life that remained to him, my father never recovered his old zest. He complained of permanent soreness in the incision area, but I am convinced the scalpel had also punctured something vital in his spirits.

I came to devour like so many novels the opaque and contradictory cancer literature—on the disease's natural development, on the outcomes of radical Prostatectomy and external-beam radiation, on less conventional treatments such as radioactive implants, cryogenic and laser surgery, and drugs. I also began phoning urologists and oncologists at teaching hospitals in North Carolina and the surrounding region. (Somewhere I had heard that physicians themselves prefer teaching institutions for second opinions and treatment when they have major medical problems.)

I discovered that all these specialists are enormously busy, but was amazed that they always returned calls, usually late the same day, having no idea who I was or what I wanted. The exception was the prominent surgeon mentioned earlier, whose assistant called instead. That man's urgent warning was the most unsettling of my conversations, and subsequent experts told me it was nonsense. Still, most counseled against delay. Said one, "Don't try to intellectualize this thing—get rid of it. You can't cure yourself. You'll just have to become a patient."

BUT BY THEN I had learned enough to be uncomfortable with this counsel. Among the articles Jane turned up, for instance, was a 1988 survey of 304 urologists and oncologists in Canada, the U.S., and Britain, asking each what treatment he would choose if he were 67 and diagnosed with gland-confined, moderately differentiated prostate cancer—close to my situation, except for age.

From the replies, it's clear the specialists preach what they practice: 79% of the U.S. urologists (most of whom are trained in surgery) said they would take radical Prostatectomy, while 92% of radiation oncologists preferred radiation. Of the urologists from Britain, where radical prostatectomies are a comparative rarity, only 4% wanted surgery, 44% opted for radiation, and the rest chose "watchful waiting," which amounts to no treatment at all until the cancer shows signs of having spread, at which point hormone therapy is given.

The U.S. is practically alone in its enthusiasm for aggressive treatment, despite conflicting evidence as to whether it does much good. In 1990 physicians from a Veterans Administration hospital and the University of Wisconsin published results of their 15-year follow-up of 111 patients with early prostate cancer. With the patients' prior consent, the physicians had randomly assigned half of them to have surgery and half to receive only a placebo. After 15 years, in the 95 patients whose history they could trace, the researchers found no significant differences in cancer mortality between the two groups and, in fact, no overall mortality difference between the cancer patients and the male population in general.

Owing partly perhaps to the prevalence of national health systems in Europe, where bureaucrats might be expected to take cost-benefit approaches to expensive remedies of questionable worth, the watchful-waiting approach is much more favored there. In 1992 a Swedish study reported ten-year outcomes of 223 early-stage prostate cancer patients who went untreated until cancer spread was evident. At that point they got hormone therapy. Again, the untreated group fared about as well as the treated. At the end of ten years, 8.5% had died of prostate cancer and 47% had died of other causes. Their overall mortality rate didn't differ significantly from that of another group that received radiation—or from the average for all Swedish men.

In the U.S., as urologists learned the nerve-sparing surgery technique - and patients heard about it—the number of radical prostatectomies jumped nearly sixfold between 1984 and 1990, while radiation treatments increased by 50%. Still, even U.S. urologists differ capriciously in recommending radical Prostatectomy, their specialty. A recent survey of Medicare records turned up the fascinating fact that if you're a patient on the West Coast, you're 3 1/2 times more likely to have prostate surgery than if you're from New England (and if you're in Washington State, 16 times more likely than in Rhode Island). The North Carolina surgery rate is closer to the Pacific Coast's than to New England's. When experts disagree to this extent, the patient has to make some choices.

In talking with physicians in my region, I found plenty of discussion of surgery and radiation but little willingness to consider watchful waiting. One exception was Jonathan Jarow, a urologist at Wake Forest University's Bowman Gray Medical Center in Winston-Salem. Jarow trained at Johns Hopkins under Patrick Walsh, the noted developer of the nerve-sparing surgical technique. Even so, before I had broached the subject in our first phone conversation, Jarow mentioned the controversy over aggressive treatment that had been raised by the Swedish studies and said that Willet Whitmore, retired head of urology at New York City's Memorial Sloan-Kettering Cancer Institute, was a leading proponent of the watchful-waiting, or "conservative," approach.

Around this time, I suggested to FORTUNE that a patient's-eye view of the prostate-cancer treatment dilemma might interest the magazine's readers. After getting a go-ahead, I began interviewing far afield, starting with Willet Whitmore.

A cordial, avuncular man of 75, Whitmore is widely regarded as an elder statesman of the urological world. Among other things, he devised the widely used criteria for classifying prostate cancers into stages—A, B, C, and D—according to tumor size, prevalence, and metastatic state. He has also condensed the essential quandary of the field into what's widely referred to as "Whitmore's Question," to wit: "Is a cure possible in those for whom it is necessary, and is a cure necessary in those for whom it is possible?"

Autopsies and surveys show that more than a third of all men over 50 already have at least microscopic malignant prostate tumors. About 13% will eventually develop diagnosable cancers, and some 3% will eventually die of them. The low death rate results more from the characteristically slow growth of most prostate cancers than from medical countermeasures. "Growing old is invariably fatal," Whitmore says, "while prostate cancer is only sometimes so."

Whitmore has been reanalyzing and combining data from many surveys of treatment outcomes. Historically, about half of the surgical and radiation treatments have turned out to be too late, since the cancer had already metastasized. That fact was largely attributable to the notorious unreliability of the digital-rectal exam, which more often than not fails to recognize tumors before they spread. Presumably, the new detection methods should improve that record, but evidence for this is so far lacking.

Moreover, says Whitmore, prostate cancer's slow growth implies that newly diagnosed men over 70 stand a good chance of dying of something else. "But if the patient is a young man," he adds, "I'd advise him to have treatment, and since I'm a surgeon, I'm inclined to advise surgery." Still, much of the recent boom in surgery is in older patients, often at their insistence.

Taken at face value, Whitmore's analyses seem to show a small survival advantage for surgery over watchful waiting and a larger advantage over radiation, but he says most of the surveys are biased in various ways. Much of the superiority claimed for prostatectomies, for instance, reflects the fact that candidates for surgery have traditionally tended to be the youngest and healthiest patients. Also, surgery furnishes an opportunity to examine nearby tissue and lymph nodes for metastasis before proceeding, so radiation and watchful waiting wind up with surgery's rejects.

Across the board, Whitmore calculates, a radical Prostatectomy might conceivably add as much as a year more to the average patient's life expectancy than the conservative approach. "Nobody argues that aggressive treatment makes a major contribution to lifespan," he says, "but it can damage life quality. In calculating the tradeoff between quality in the near term against an added year at a time when quality may not be all that great, the patient has to apply his own discount rate. It's his decision."

GERALD CHODAK, co-director of urologic oncology at the University of Chicago medical school and a surgeon himself, finds other biases at work in most surveys, which tend to overstate the benefits of aggressive treatment. He notes, for instance, that improved diagnostics and earlier treatment have increased the survival times reported for individual patients. Yet the overall mortality rates for all prostate cancer victims has not improved. How can that be? The answer, Chodak points out, is that survival is counted from the time of diagnosis, so with earlier diagnosis, more time elapses before death. But death often occurs no later than it would have without treatment.

Furthermore, the new diagnostic measures turn up many small tumors that probably wouldn't prove fatal if left untreated, so the treatment's apparent benefits are illusory. Chodak is a foremost critic of recent proposals for a national program to screen men for prostate cancer. Depending upon the methods used, a one-time screening of all men over 50 could cost $7 billion to $28 billion. Even the smaller figure exceeds the entire federal cancer budget.

SINCE THE 1950s, the prevailing explanation for the unpredictability of prostate cancer is that at least two species exist—a very slow-growing "indolent" type and a very fast-growing "aggressive" type. In this view, the main challenge for research is learning how to distinguish between them. Absent that ability, many argue, prudence dictates getting rid of all tumors thought to be still confined to the prostate.

But another school of thought, centered around pathologist John McNeal and urologist Thomas Stamey, both at the Stanford medical school, contends that all prostate tumors are basically the same, following the same natural history and changing character in predictable ways. McNeal developed this theory in the course of slicing into thin sections some 600 preserved prostates removed at Stanford over the years. He calculated the volume of each cancer by adding up the tumor areas in each slice. He correlated those results with evidence of metastases in the glands' former possessors. He concluded that tumor size alone is a fair gauge of malignancy, for as cancer cells divide they undergo a series of mutations that increase their aggressive behavior and may lead them to escape from the prostate.

McNeal says that malignant tumors measuring less than half a cubic centimeter—about the size of a pea—are found in about 32% of white men and 45% of black men over 50; the tumors double in size about every three to four years. In all but the youngest patients, these may be regarded as essentially harmless since they will take so long to reach metastatic size. He estimates that a four-cubic-centimeter tumor—as big as a large marble—has only a 10% probability of having already spread at the time of discovery. But if the cancer is not found until it measures ten cubic centimeters, it has almost certainly escaped.

The problem lies in measuring tumors in living patients. The traditional digital-rectal exam is far too unreliable, and even ultrasound doesn't provide adequate images. The Stanford approach relies on inserting six or more biopsy needles into the prostate in a carefully spaced array. From the number of needles that encounter a tumor and the length of the malignant tissue in the extracted cores, pathologists can make a fair estimate of size.

The Stanford group goes on to claim that once the size of a tumor is estimated and its Gleason grade determined, periodic PSA measurements will reliably indicate its rate of growth, providing a rough measure of its predilection to spread. That resolves the fundamental conundrum of the watchful-waiting approach—what to watch.

There's plenty of dispute about various aspects of the Stanford theory. Jonathan Epstein, a prominent Johns Hopkins pathologist, says he has evidence that even small tumors occasionally metastasize. McNeal doesn't entirely discount that possibility but doesn't think it very likely. Other experts contend that PSA levels fluctuate too much to be relied upon, but McNeal says that thousands of Stanford blood tests demonstrate PSA to be a reliable reflection of tumor growth unless temporarily elevated by stresses from infection, biopsies, or digital-rectal exams.

By this time, I thought I had part of the answer to Whitmore's question. Because of my age, health, and good fortune in having found the cancer early, a cure was probably possible. What wasn't so clear was whether it was necessary. Having talked with several other men who had wrestled or were wrestling with the same question, I was impressed by how personal that decision is. The others I knew had opted for treatment on the reasonable ground that at the very least it was a form of insurance. A major contributor to quality of life, after all, is the assurance that one is rid of a cancer.

Apart from my own natural reluctance to risk the debilities of treatment at this period of my life, though, I felt that with the field of prostate cancer management in such flux and with new, minimally invasive treatment approaches—medications, new techniques for destroying tumors by freezing, and so forth—now building a record, I'd prefer to postpone doing anything if I prudently could. According to Chicago's Gerald Chodak, I stand about an 87% chance of not dying of cancer in the next ten years—considerably better than the odds against my dying of other ailments—though the odds against metastasis are only about 60%. But even with immediate treatment, Chodak puts the likelihood of metastasis at 20% to 30% and my odds of dying from prostate cancer within a decade at 6% or 7%. "What you do," he says, "largely depends on your anxiety level."

SHORTLY AFTERWARD, I got wind of some major studies to be published in late May in the Journal of the American Medical Association by teams of researchers from several universities working on a federally sponsored prostate cancer project. When I made contact with the group, Dartmouth's John Wasson faxed me summaries that had already been delivered to professional gatherings. What most interested me was a computer model the project had developed to compare the benefits and risks of surgery, radiation, and watchful waiting for patients of different ages and tumor grades.

Taking the case of a man of 65 in good to excellent health with a localized, moderately differentiated tumor—the example closest to my own situation—the model predicts an expected life of 13.3 years with watchful waiting. Depending upon his estimate of treatment effectiveness, he might expect to live 13.6 to 14 years after radical surgery and 13.7 to 14.1 years after external-beam radiation. But if the patient adjusted those future years for quality by setting a year of impotence to be worth only 95%, for example, and took a few other variables into account, the model predicts that he would generally find himself better off with watchful waiting.

By then nearly five months had elapsed since my first PSA test. I still hadn't selected a physician I felt comfortable with—one who seemed at ease with the notion of watchful waiting. I finally called Jonathan Jarow at Bowman Gray in Winston-Salem and asked him what he thought about such a course. He frankly replied that I was the first patient who had ever asked him that. "Most want to get rid of the stuff as quickly as possible," he said. He admitted to knowing little about the approach, but he agreed to see me and talk about it.

On our first meeting, I was even more favorably impressed than on the telephone. Jarow, 36, seemed open and interested, while cross-examining me pretty closely on what I thought I wanted to do and why. But he added that since our conversation he had attended an American Urological Association meeting, where he had talked to others about my situation. He sensed a shift of opinion in the profession toward more conservative approaches. He also ordered up a blood test. Five days later, he called with the results: My PSA reading was up to 10.2—from 5.9 only five months before. I knew enough by then to be stunned. Though I had expected some increase, by the Stanford logic my tumor appeared to have grown by more than half, suggesting a doubling time of less than a year—and obvious urgency about getting something done. Clearly troubled himself, Jarow proposed another PSA test in a few weeks' time. I missed some sleep again.

Continuing my research, though, I raised the issue of sudden PSA jumps in interviews with several experts, including John McNeal of Stanford and Patrick Walsh of Johns Hopkins. Both thought something was amiss—perhaps a lab mix-up on the first or second test, perhaps an infection of some sort.

Knowing Jarow to be an old Johns Hopkins man, I was hesitant to broach the Stanford theory when I reported to Bowman Gray for my next test. But he readily agreed that if the next PSA reading was down, we'd try a multi-needle biopsy. (I later discovered that Epstein and others at Johns Hopkins now advocate a pattern-biopsy approach similar to Stanford's, though they tend to emphasize Gleason grade more than size.)

As it turned out, this time my PSA was down to 6.9. On entering the Bowman Gray ultrasound room on August 9 and seeing the long row of small jars lined up to receive my tissue samples, I knew I was in for an ordeal. I lay on my left side, facing away from Jarow and his machine. At his suggestion, I had brought along a small mirror to watch the ultrasound screen as he did a quick scan of my prostate—not that I could make much sense of the grainy smudges that drifted about the screen as he twisted and turned the probe. Early on, Jarow announced that he could see no clear signs of any tumor, but he quickly quashed any emergent hope by adding that ultrasound was simply not very good at doing that.

Then he cocked the biopsy gun and began extracting samples, spaced half a centimeter apart across the length and breadth of the gland. The patient feels about what one might expect—sharp stings, each seemingly worse than the last, as bits of nerve-bearing tissue are snatched from his interior. By the time the 15 samples were taken, sweat was pouring from my forehead and I was happy for the process to end.

ON THE EVENING of Friday the 13th, Jarow called with the pathologist's report. Of the 15 biopsy cores, two adjacent ones near the rear tip of the gland contained small amounts of tumor tissue. The pathologist had assigned one a Gleason score of 3+3, but the other contained too little malignant material to score at all. Typical of the ambiguity in prostate cancer diagnostics, the one-point jump in Gleason score since my previous biopsy could signal tumor progression—but could also merely represent a different sampling site or a different pathologist's judgment. Assuming both cores to be from the same tumor, it presumably has a volume between 0.5 and 1.5 cubic centimeters.

At this point, Jarow and I resumed our gentle debate over what to do next, he playing devil's advocate to my own predilection for deferring treatment. He pointed out that all the theories about predicting tumor behavior - from Stanford, Johns Hopkins, wherever —are rooted in ex post facto attempts to tie observations of prostates removed at one point in time to metastases that took place at some earlier juncture, without knowing when the metastases actually occurred. Hence all that the theories can really determine is when it's probably too late for a cure.

My position, admittedly influenced by Stanford's 600 prostate dissections, was that I didn't expect certainty, but that if 90% of the patients without metastases had tumors smaller than four cubic centimeters at the time of surgery, then most metastases must happen after tumors get larger than that. I could live with monitoring my tumor's growth for some time yet while also watching for upward shifts in Gleason grade and PSA.

AS A FINAL PROBE of my position, Jarow wondered whether I would really be happy living from test to test that way. If I chose watchful waiting, wouldn't it be better to make the decision final and have no more tests until metastasis occurred, at which point I would go on hormone therapy? I replied that I wasn't yet prepared to go that far. Having tests doesn't make me as anxious as not having them, and maybe something will come along - new knowledge, new therapies, perhaps—to change my mind about treatment.

We concluded by agreeing on a plan: In nine months I will get another blood test. If my PSA level at that point is around 7 or below, we'll do nothing except continue tracking PSA. If the level has risen to between 7 and 10, I'll have another biopsy to look for substantial increases in my tumor's size or grade. If either is evident—or if my PSA reads much above 10—I'll reconsider treatment.

By now I've learned that Jarow likes to have trigger points for future action neatly pinned down this way, but he also has a surprising open-mindedness about what the plan should be. At the close of a recent consultation, Jane asked him what he would do if he were a prostate-cancer victim like me - a question I hadn't bothered asking, since I thought I knew what this surgeon would say. But I was wrong. "I honestly don't know," he replied. Which in some odd way was enormously comforting.

Fortune Magazine
May 13, 1996

STILL WAITING, WATCHFULLY
By
Tom Alexander

I get a lot of calls and letters nowadays from people wondering, I suspect, whether I'm dead yet. In September 1993, I wrote an article for Fortune chronicling my prostate cancer diagnosis and my struggle to decide what to do about it. In brief, it appeared that I had a relatively small tumor and that my options were surgery or radiation. My urologist estimated the odds of a successful cure at about 95% for surgery and 75% to 85% for radiation, and also warned that if I didn't do something, chances were 40% that the tumor would metastasize within five years and therefore be incurable.

In subsequent second opinions and my own research, I discovered growing controversy about these numbers, including some evidence that the physician may have overstated the prospects of success and understated the likelihood of untoward consequences of these accepted treatments. According to some surveys of patients who'd had radical prostatectomies, about 50% became incontinent and 88% experienced impotence. As I wound my way through the contradictory medical literature and interviewed experts, I became aware that, in fact, there was dispute over whether any of the known treatments was likely to prolong my life or, if it did, whether the prospective few weeks or months that might be added to the end of my life would outweigh the potential damage to life's quality, starting now.

With some initially hesitant support from a frightfully young urologist, Jonathan Jarow, at Bowman Gray Medical Center in Winston-Salem, North Carolina, I decided on watchful waiting, which amounts to doing nothing except monitoring my disease. What I didn't know at the time was that I was joining an enormous cohort of scared and bewildered men whose long-unsuspected tumors had only then been uncovered by the powerful new blood test for "prostate specific antigen" or PSA. As soon as my article appeared, I began receiving letters and phone calls from other newly diagnosed men. Since no information had been given about where I lived, except for a vague reference in the article to "western North Carolina," they had exerted ingenuity to locate my address or phone number.

Early on, from what I was hearing, most urologists were strongly urging immediate surgery on my callers and correspondents - no matter what their situation. I suspect that the majority of men in my situation do get treatment. Many indicate that they're under strong pressure not only from their physicians but from their wives and families to get that stuff out of there. I count myself lucky in having a wife, Jane, who has never questioned my decision and in having a physician, Jarow, who often seems even more skeptical of treatment than I.

Though trained in radical Prostatectomy at Johns Hopkins by Patrick Walsh, who is widely regarded as the best in the business, Jarow contends that the men most likely to be cured - those with the small, low-grade tumors that surgeons like and that PSA tests now pick up in abundance - may not need curing since they'll probably live to die of something else. On the other hand, he says, men who most need to be cured - those with large, advanced tumors - probably can't be cured, since their cancer is likely already out of the barn.

Since I wrote the article, it appears that more physicians currently accept watchful waiting as a legitimate option in the case of small, low-to moderate-grade prostate tumors, even in "young" men such as myself (I'm 65). A team from the Mayo Clinic, for example, has defined as "clinically insignificant" most prostate tumors unlikely to grow larger than 20 cubic centimeters in the projected lifetime of the patient.

My waiting strategy relies on PSA as a surrogate for changes in tumor volume and malignancy, which in turn are supposed to warn when my cancer may start to grow rapidly. A normal PSA is usually considered anything below 4 nanograms per milliliter of blood. At diagnosis my level was 5.9 but it has since soared as high as 10.9 possibly because of an infection, and dipped as low as 5.8. Besides PSA fluctuations, another difficulty, which Jarow is careful to point out, is that by the time we've seen a PSA move convincing enough to act upon, it may be too late.

I still keep treatment as a fallback in case things look as if they're turning sour. For the moment, though, I have no symptoms and I find living with prostate cancer gets easier all the time. The actual morality and even the relative risk are, after all, not very different from auto fatalities, but who hesitates to jump into a car for a movie? I probably wouldn't even think much about prostate cancer were it not for those calls and letters. Meanwhile, I hope for ten or fifteen years untroubled by the negative effects of either cancer or its treatments, during which time maybe some of the promising current research on genes and immunity may finally pay off with real answers to this weird disease of ours.

PERSONAL UPDATE-JAN.2000

It has now been a little over seven years since my original prostate cancer diagnosis. I've yet to undergo any real treatment or show any symptoms. Were it not for the occasional phone calls I still get from newly-diagnosed guys, in fact, I probably wouldn't think very much about prostate cancer. Most of my concerns about old age and dying nowadays tend to center around heart disease and strokes.

I still get my PSA checked about once a year, mainly at the insistence of my primary-care physician. My last PSA, in April of 1999, was 10.7, which was about double my first reading of 5.9 from December, 1992, but less than the 11.7 level of March 1998. I also swallow a bunch of food supplements whose benefits have been touted on various prostate-related Internet mailing lists that I subscribed to until I became bored with the whole subject. The ones I take include soy protein, lycopene, selenium, garlic, green tea, and multi-vitamins, plus vitamins E and C. I also take saw palmetto, which is supposed to reduce urinary frequency, as does Cardura, a prescription medication that also reduces blood pressure (which is marginally elevated in me). Whether any of these things have any effect on the progress of prostate cancer or not, I can't say with much assurance. I more or less subscribe to the chicken-soup theory: "They probably can't hoit." And they're not too expensive.

As for what lessons can be derived from my seven years' experience, I am reluctant to venture much of a guess, except to say that I don't believe the medical profession has yet to get a good handle on this bewildering disease of ours. About the strongest statement I'll make to friends who've succumbed to treatment is, "I'll bet my last seven years have been better than your last seven years." When guys call asking about watchful-waiting, I'll sometimes offer a few rules of thumb about who might reasonably contemplate such a course of (in) action; namely,

1. An age greater than 60 at time of diagnosis,
2. A PSA doubling time of more than four years,
3. A Gleason score of 6 (3+3) or less,
4. A single small tumor; i.e. no more than one needle showing tumor out of the normal six in the conventional sextant biopsy, and
5. Perhaps most important, a cast of mind that allows one to live with a known tumor. (Of all these rules, this one seems to be hardest for American males. Most of them I've talked to want to "get it out of there" and I have to quarrel with that.)

Implicitly, these rules are grounded in my (and others') theory that there seem to be at least two varieties of prostate cancer - an aggressive or fast-growing kind and an indolent or slow-growing kind. If you have the indolent kind, there's reasonable chance you'll die of something else (which some might say is the name of the game). On the other hand, there's some evidence that indolent disease can convert over time to the aggressive variety, which is the reason for the over 60 age limitation.

The only other thing I'd offer is that, if I WERE to go to treatment, I would probably go for the seed-implants, by one of the recognized experts in the field.

Chapter 16

PREVENTING AND CURING CANCER BY WORKING THROUGH THE MIND

Alfred A. Barrios, Ph.D.

It is now a fairly well established fact that the mind - in particular the mental state of hopelessness - can play a major role in the formation of cancer. A chronic state of hopelessness predisposes one to cancer by its suppressive effect on the immune system. If this is true, then by turning this negative state of mind around we should be able to prevent and/or eliminate any cancer present. This chapter will present strong evidence that this definitely is the case, as well as present ways of turning this hopelessness factor around.

To begin with, it should be made clear that the body does indeed have natural defenses against cancer. One of the first studies to establish this fact was presented by West (1954):

"Mass surveys that have been conducted for the detection of early cancer of the uterine cervix have produced some very enlightening information. A large group of women in whom carcinoma in situ [in its original place] was detected by the Papanicolaou technique, and later confirmed by Punch Biopsy, were followed. In only 20% of these did the malignant cells invade the basement membrane and become Grade One carcinomas requiring treatment. In the remainder this growth disturbance was self controlled and vanished. Thus, we are confronted with the very likely possibility that all of us may have had, have or will have some form of cancer. But because of inherent natural control of the neoplastic process we will never know it and will, in all probability, die of unrelated causes."

Next we need to present the evidence that a mental state of hopelessness can indeed predispose one to cancer and that if this state of hopelessness can be reversed, the immune response can be revived and the cancer prevented or rejected.

According to Temoshok in her book *The Type C Connection* (1993):

"For three decades, mind-body scientists have documented that chronic hopelessness can be damaging to our health and, specifically, to recovery from cancer. Drs. A.H. Schmale and Howard Iker from the University of Rochester studied a group of sixty-eight women before a biopsy to determine cervical cancer. The researchers were able to predict which patients had cancer with 73 percent accuracy. The single factor upon which they made their predictions was the presence of hopelessness. Karl Goodkin, M.D., and his colleagues at the University of Miami evaluated seventy-three women awaiting workup for an abnormal Pap smear. They discovered that patients with advanced disease had more life stress, and had reacted to that stress with hopelessness.

"Hopelessness has been studied in animals as well. How, you may ask, can we tell if an animal feels hopeless? While animal researchers can't exactly re-create this peculiarly human state of mind, they can create a close analogue; helplessness. The loss of control mirrors and overlaps the human experience of the loss of hope. To induce helplessness, researchers place mice in experimental situations in which they are unable to remove a source of stress - usually a shock delivered to their tails. In dozens of such studies, the helpless mice have been shown to suffer severe damage to their immune systems. Tumors implanted in these mice grow faster and cause death more rapidly."(pp.136-137).

There have also been a number of studies showing that cancer patients who were provided positive psychotherapeutic intervention aimed at, among other things, instilling a greater sense of empowerment (as opposed to helplessness-hopelessness) showed considerable improvement. This includes the work of Dr. O. Carl Simonton (1978); David Spiegel (1989) and F.I. Fawzy (1993).

Also, in support of the fact that a mental state of hopelessness plays a major role in affecting the immune system are the extensive studies of Ronald Glaser, MD and his wife psychologist Janice Kiecolt-Glaser, Ph.D. of the Ohio State College of Medicine, as reported in Norman Cousins' (1989) book *Head First: The Biology of Hope*:

The Glaser\Kiecolt-Glaser team observed immune impairment in individuals enduring chronic (unrelenting) stress (leading to a state of chronic hopelessness). In one study thirty-four caregivers of Alzheimer's disease victims were compared with thirty-four control subjects. Caregivers had lower percentages of total T-cells, helper T-cells and helper\suppressor T-cell ratios and higher antibody titers to latent viruses (all various aspects of the immune response). In another study Drs. Kiecolt-Glaser and Glaser compared thirty eight married and thirty eight separated or divorced women. The researchers found that women who had been separated or divorced were more depressed, and had lower percentages of NK cells, less immune stimulability, and higher antibody titers to latent viruses.

The Glasers have also demonstrated that the reduction of stress or the enhancement of positive emotions (including hopefulness) can have the effect of boosting immunity. For instance when the above mentioned Alzheimer's caregivers were placed in a support group, they felt substantially less lonely and had significantly higher percentages of NK cells than those not involved in a support group.

Other studies showing that psychotherapeutic interventions can enhance the immune response include those of Dr. Haberman and Levy of the Pittsburgh Cancer Institute - another immunologist and psychologist team. Along with psychologists Judith Rodin and Martin Seligman, they conducted a pilot study of patients with melanoma and colon cancer to see if psychological treatment could boost the patients' natural immunity. Of the thirty patients in the study all received standard medical treatment, but half were given an eight-week course in relaxation techniques and cognitive therapy. The relaxation helped the patients reduce stress and the cognitive therapy helped them to cope with depression, regain control, and cultivate optimism (the opposite of hopelessness). In his book, *Learned Optimism*. Dr. Seligman describes Sandra Levy's reaction when she got the first definitive results from their study:

"Holy Cow! You should have seen those numbers". I have never heard Sandy as excited as she was on the phone that November morning, two years later. "The natural killer cell activity is up very sharply in the cancer patients who got cognitive therapy. Not at all in the controls. Holy Cow!" In short, cognitive therapy strongly enhanced immune activity-just as we hoped it would (p.203).

Not only did the therapy patients have stronger NK cells, but they were less depressed and self-blaming.

As pointed out in the chapter on cancer and the mind in my book *Towards Greater Freedom and Happiness* (1985), there are two basic types of hopelessness that can play a part in cancer. The first type of hopelessness results from the often "death sentence" interpretation of a cancer diagnosis. The second type of hopelessness that is often also present in cancer patients is a deeply embedded hopelessness about life in general. And, as Temoshok puts it, not only is this second type of hopelessness often present in cancer patients but what makes things even more hopeless is that the person "has no faith that things can ever change":

"Hopelessness is both a mind state and, if you will, a non-belief system. A person who feels hopeless may go about business as usual, but inside he has given up on life's possibilities. He finds that his needs - psychological, spiritual, creative - have been frustrated and, in his view, will remain that way into the distant future. What is significant is not that he feels trapped, unfulfilled, and abandoned, it's that he feels trapped, unfulfilled, abandoned and *has no faith that things can ever change.*

"The cancer patient is prone to two shades of hopelessness. She may suddenly look back on her life and realize I've never had a full sense of meaning and joy in my work and relationships, and I never will. The other shade relates to the fight against cancer. The person says, There's nothing I can do to help myself get better, I'm never going to recover." (Temoshok, 1993, p.136)

What then, is the best approach to eliminating both types of hopelessness?

I. In order to eliminate the "death-sentence-diagnosis-of-cancer type of hopelessness I first present the evidence that the body has natural defense mechanism against cancer. Thus if you can reverse the negative mental state of hopelessness which has been shown to suppress this natural defense mechanism then you can reverse the cancer (see above). I follow this by presenting a number of testimonials - case histories of patients that have been successfully cured using this mind-body approach. Hearing about actual case histories where the mind-body approach has worked will further increase the hope/belief factor. Some excellent examples can be found in chapter 13 (Stories of Hope, Change, and Survival) of Temoshok's (1993) book. Take for instance the story of Irwin. Diagnosed initially with testicular cancer, the cancer had eventually spread to his lymph nodes, chest and lungs. One tumor on his neck had grown so large he was forced to keep his head at an odd tilt. His doctors told him that even with the best treatment at the time (a combination of surgery, radiation, cobalt and nitrogen mustard) he had only three to four months to live and that he had zero chance of survival. At this point he sought the help of a psychotherapist who used hypnosis along with traditional psychoanalysis. Under hypnosis he was much more open to healing suggestions aimed at overcoming blocks in his capacity to love and be loved and to work on achieving his long term life goals. Within six months, he had resolved his love problems and gotten married, and was ordained as an Episcopal priest - a lifelong goal. On the very day he was ordained he got the news that his follow-up x-rays showed no more evidence of cancer. His lymph nodes and lungs were completely clear. Today, *thirty-three years later*, Irwin is alive, well and cancer-free.

Other equally exciting case histories can be found in my book *Towards Greater Freedom and Happiness* (1985, pp.151-153) or on my website, www.stresscards.com in the Dr. Barrios articles section - the article on cancer.

II. Eliminating the second type of hopelessness in cancer patients - the hopelessness about their life in general - is usually a bit more difficult. This is because, as Temoshok (1993) points out, it is usually very difficult for people to change deeply embedded life-long attitudes, beliefs and habits. She gives many examples of such difficulty throughout her book:

"Despite these realizations, Naomi said that changing her old behavior was one of the hardest things she'd ever attempted" (p.28).

"Through the course of my research, I learned that some people cannot change their Type C [cancer prone] behavior, for reasons that were hard to discern" (p.44).

"I never wanted to be unhappy, to deny my feelings, to let people take advantage of me, and I certainly never wanted to get sick! I was stuck, and now realize how deep-seated it was and how hard it is to change"(p.219).

"What about our immune systems and the mind-body factors that influence our health? Don't we have control over them? Treya had come to realize we don't have total control even over these internal factors. As I said, the Type C pattern is not a path that anyone consciously chooses, and changing it can be difficult. We don't have complete mastery over our feelings and behavior" (p.223).

Incidentally, these quotes can give us insight into how to deal with a current problem associated with the mind-body approach to cancer. The problem is that many people are made to feel guilty, because this approach implies that we consciously caused the negative behavior that led to our cancer; if this is so, then we should easily be able to change this negative behavior. As can be seen by what Temoshok has said, not only have we not consciously chosen to instill all this cancer causing negative behavior, but also most people (without effective psychotherapy) do not have much conscious control over changing this behavior.

The solution I have come up with to effectively deal with this difficulty-of-change problem is a program called Self-Programmed Control or SPC which uses a unique combination of hypnosis and biofeedback techniques to facilitate re-programming of the underlying negative behavior. To give you some idea of how much more effective hypnotherapy is compared to other forms of psychotherapy, I refer you to my article entitled: Hypnotherapy: A reappraisal (Barrios, 1970) where the following statistics were presented:

"Comparing the results of several studies...we find that for psychoanalysis we can expect a recovery rate of 38% after approximately 600 sessions.

For Wolpian therapy [Behavior Therapy], we can expect a recovery rate of 72% after an average of 22 sessions, and for hypnotherapy we can expect a recovery rate of 93% after an average of 6 sessions".

It is interesting to note the negative correlation between the number of sessions and the percentage recovery rate. At first this seems paradoxical. However, if a form of therapy is truly effective, it should not only increase recovery rate, but also shorten the number of sessions necessary (as well as widen the range of cases treatable.)

It might help the reader to understand why hypnosis is such a powerful tool for facilitating change, if one understands that hypnosis can best be defined as a state of heightened belief (Barrios, 1969). As it has been pointed out in Chapter I of *Towards Greater Freedom and Happiness* (Barrios, 1985), we know how important a part belief can play in facilitating reprogramming and thus in being able to change (reprogram) deeply imbedded involuntary or automatic behavior.

Currently we seem to know a lot about programming and reprogramming computers, but when it comes to the main computer - the human brain - we still seem to be in the dark ages. But SPC, with its highly effective (self) hypnotic techniques, is the ray of light that can help us out of this darkness.

One final comment: You should be aware that not all hypnosis is the same. Some techniques are more effective than others for increasing the all powerful belief factor. It is felt that because of the inherent immediate positive feedback (belief building) aspects of the SPC techniques, SPC is one of the more effective hypnotherapeutic approaches.

Reprogramming The Negative

In order to reprogram the negative attitudes, beliefs and habits that are causing the overall general state of hopelessness one must not only first have a good idea of what they are, but also what to program in their place. The book *Towards Greater Freedom and Happiness* will be your guide for both. Each individual will find certain areas of the book that are especially pertinent for him and of course these areas should be focused on most.

Further Considerations

There are many in the medical community who might be fearful that the mind-body approach might convince cancer patients to forgo the standard medical treatments. Is there any justification for this fear? Are we saying that with the mind-body approach there is no need for any physical treatments? The answer, of course, is no. If we look upon an established cancer as self-perpetuating, as a carcinogenic agent itself, so to speak, then we would want to do anything within reason to remove this carcinogenic agent - just as we would want to remove a person from over-exposure to radiation, asbestos, cigarette smoke, etc. However, we also have to take into account the possible iatrogenic (doctor-caused illness) qualities of the standard treatments. It is a known fact that chemotherapy and radiation therapy, while eliminating the primary cancer, are immuno-suppressive and as a result may very well lead to secondary cancers (Penn, 1974; Selby, 1985). Also, there are certain surgical procedures that can lead to secondary cancers indirectly due to depressive effects of disfigurement (e.g. breast removal) or impairment (e.g. impotence resulting from removal of the prostate).

What would be ideal, would be to use less toxic forms of treatment in conjunction with a mind-body approach such as SPC. This could include such methods as the new prostate radioactive seed implantation approach (see chapter on seed implant therapy in this book) where the potential damage of radiation to surrounding healthy tissue is considerably less than that in standard radiation treatment. (Incidentally, it was a combination of both SPC and Prostate Seed Implantation that Michael O'Hara chose to follow, and last time I checked he was doing great).

Another less toxic approach that can be combined with SPC is hyperthermia, which uses focused heat in combination with low dosages of radiation to kill the tumors. (See *Consensus on Hyperthermia for the 1990's* edited by Bicher & Hastal, 1990, where they report considerable success with prostate cancer.)

And, of course, anyone opting for the wait and see approach currently popular with many prostate cancer patients would be wise to combine this with the SPC approach.

REFERENCES

All the articles and books referenced in this chapter can be found in the reference section of the Cancer and The Mind article at my website, www.stresscards.com, in the articles section.

Chapter 17

THE BENEFITS OF COMMUNITY BASED CANCER SUPPORT PROGRAMS - USING THE WELLNESS COMMUNITY AS AN EXAMPLE

By
Harold H. Benjamin, Ph.D. (c) 2000
Founder, The Wellness Community

It has long been believed that when cancer is the diagnosis, death is a certainty and that the patient is relegated to being hopeless, helpless and passive—that there is nothing he or she can do to be a part of the fight for recovery. This is not true. According to the American Cancer Society, "when adjusted for normal life expectancy, a relative five year survival rate of 58% is seen for all cancers, and there are more than 8,000,000 Americans alive today who have a history of cancer." Additionally, the myth that the cancer patient is hopeless, helpless and passive in the face of the illness is being dispelled more each day.

Scientists are rapidly learning that there is much cancer patients can do to join with their physician in the fight for recovery and that their participation may have a positive effect on the course of the illness. However, although these facts have been known to scientists for several years, they are not well known to the general public.

As an answer to that problem, in 1982, The Wellness Community was formed as a program where cancer patients and their families could, without cost, learn and practice the techniques of being a "Patient Active". That's the designation we use at The Wellness Community to describe a cancer patient who has decided to join with his or her physician in the fight for recovery. Since then, other community and hospital based Cancer Support Programs have emerged. There are those who call the period of time starting with The Wellness Community "The Patient Active Era" - acknowledging that the patient can play a conscious, purposeful part in their fight for recovery if he or she wants to.

Regarding the Patient Active Concept, The Wellness Community is now the largest Cancer Support Program in the world, with 20 facilities nation-wide, now seeing over 5,000 participants each week. We have provided psychosocial support to more than 45,000 participants since opening and hundreds of oncologists are on our Professional Advisory Boards. Everyone who interacts with participants at The Wellness Community is a licensed psychotherapist and there is never any cost to the participant.

The Wellness Community and other Cancer Support Programs are on the cutting edge of a Cultural Revolution in health care "The Patient Active Era". It is my prediction that by the year 2030/2040 a Cultural Revolution will have evolved to where "The Patient Active Concept" its methods and techniques, as provided by The Wellness Community, will have become part of the common wisdom throughout the U.S., and that physicians will take the psychological temperature of the patient as routinely as he or she takes the physical temperature.

The following statements, basic to The Wellness Community, will set forth the context in which our program is offered and will describe the new position of the patient as a partner in the fight for recovery.

* Cancer patients who join with their physicians in the fight for recovery will improve the quality of their lives and may enhance the possibility of recovery. (The Patient Active Concept)
* The Wellness Community combines the Will of the patient and the Skill of the physician, a mighty combination.
* The Wellness Community makes many suggestions as to the fight for recovery. If you do all of them or none of them - that's the right thing for you. You are the perfect you.
* The Wellness Community Program and the Patient Active Concept are suggestions only. There are no absolutes.
* There is a fine line to walk. On the one hand, you should know that there are actions you can take to join with your

physician in the fight for recovery and that your participation may have a positive effect on the course of the illness. On the other hand, it must be absolutely clear that there is not even the inference or implication that if you enter the fight things are certain to turn out as you want them to. Biology often overcomes psychology.

* The Wellness Community Program is in support of and an integral part of conventional medical treatment, not an alternative.

  Before describing the Program, it will be helpful for you to know a few basic facts about cancer, reduced to its most simple form, to understand why our suggestions may be helpful.
* Cancer cells appear in most of our bodies from time to time.
* The reason we don't all develop cancer is because most of the time our immune system is strong enough to destroy the cancer cells when they appear.
* If cancer is the diagnosis it means that the cancer cells have appeared and the immune system was not strong enough to handle them
* Long term, unremitting, unpleasant emotions, usually called stress, depress the immune system and pleasant emotions enhance the immune system.
* After cancer has been diagnosed, if pleasant emotions are enhanced and stress is reduced, the immune system will become stronger, thereby, perhaps, enhancing the possibility of recovery.
* The individual has some control over his or her reactions to life events - the amount of stress he or she undergoes.

It is our hope and expectation that by participating in a Cancer Support Program, cancer patients will learn methods and techniques to maximize pleasant emotions and minimize stress, which can lead to improving their quality of life and the possibility of recovery. With this in mind, The Wellness Community provides cancer patients and their families the following programs:

GENERAL STATEMENT: The Wellness Community is, above everything else, a community - a homelike place where people with cancer and their families can come together to build support and a sense of extended family, reducing feelings of unwanted aloneness. It is a place where they can come to attain the knowledge needed, on the psychological and emotional level, to fight for recovery along with their medical team. Every aspect of The Wellness Community free program, listed below, is to help cancer patients improve the quality of their lives and fight for recovery.

HOMELIKE FACILITY AVAILABLE ALL DAY: At The Wellness Community, cancer patients learn about the unique "Patient Active Concept," which combines the will of the patient and the skill of the physician. They meet and learn from their physician and each other, they can involve themselves in the fight. All participants are invited to use the community in much the same way as they would use a neighborhood center. Participants and staff are present throughout the day and there are evening and weekend activities.

ORIENTATION MEETINGS: Two times a week informal drop-in groups are led by cancer survivors. At these meetings, people with cancer learn that their diagnosis is not always a death sentence, that life does not end with the diagnosis, that they can learn ways to participate in their fight for recovery along with their physician and that there is hope - always hope. It is at these meetings that they learn about the wide variety of Wellness Community programs and services available for their use.

PATIENT ACTIVE SUPPORT GROUPS: These are on-going two-hour weekly support groups led by licensed psychotherapists specially trained in TWC's methods of dealing with the psychological and emotional problems of cancer patients. In these groups, participants (1) become part of an extended family of those who understand, (2) learn new and different methods for dealing with the physical and emotional problems associated with the illness, and (3) perhaps relieve some of the stress in their lives. Participant groups are for people with cancer who are actively fighting for physical recovery and are willing to make a weekly commitment.*

PATIENT ACTIVE FAMILY GROUPS: Similar to participant groups, these are ongoing two-hour weekly support groups led by licensed psychotherapists specially trained in TWC's methods of dealing with the psychological and emotional problems that caregivers face when a loved one is diagnosed with cancer. In these groups, caregivers learn how best to support the person with cancer, while supporting themselves - much to the benefit of both.

RELAXATION/VISUALIZATION: Participants practice a physical relaxation exercise in order to attain the "relaxation response" combined with a visualization or guided-imagery experience. Harold H. Benjamin, Ph.D. in The Wellness Community Guide to Fighting for Recovery from Cancer, citing the work of Herbert Benson, MD and O. Carl Simonton, MD, discusses the importance of combining these two components as a tool in the fight for recovery. R/V is often helpful for people dealing with pain, side effects of chemotherapy, radiation treatment and reducing stress.

EDUCATIONAL WORKSHOPS: Several times each month, workshops, lectures and seminars are conducted by prominent physicians, oncologists, psychologists and other professionals that provide information and education useful for people with cancer. "Ask The Physician," Nutrition Workshops and Exercise Programs are examples of these drop-in groups. Of course, TWC does not advocate any position in these presentations.

NETWORKING GROUPS FOR SPECIFIC TYPES OF CANCER: These groups are facilitated focus groups, meeting regularly, where people with specific types of cancer meet, discuss and exchange information about their specific cancer. Breast Cancer

Networking Group and The Prostate Cancer Group are two examples of this type of program.

COMMUNITY EVENTS: There are social gatherings, such as parties, potlucks, game nights, joke tests, sing-alongs and other celebratory events, which brings participants, family members and friends together to laugh and play.

I reiterate that all of the above is provided in the hope and expectation that if the cancer patient participates in their fight for recovery, he or she will improve their quality of life and may enhance the possibility of recovery in their fight for recovery.

For more or further information about The Wellness Community and other Cancer Support Communities please call 310 314 2555.

SECTION III

REAL EXPERIENCES FROM REAL PEOPLE

Chapter 18

PROSTATE PROBLEMS AREN'T ALWAYS ABOUT CANCER

by William Toomey, Gold Medal Winning Olympic Decathlete.

Prostate Cancer is not the only problem that male Americans have to deal with. There are a variety of prostate disorders that afflict us, and too often, we languish hoping it will go away.

Why is it we don't seek help? The unfortunate part of these problems under the heading of BENIGN PROSTATIC HYPERPLASIA (BPH), is that the condition develops on a cell by cell basis, and its growth is so subtle, that it is barely noticeable. 60% of men between the ages of 40 and 60 years already have an enlarged prostate!

We deal with BPH by ignoring it until around the age of 50 when the symptoms become uncomfortable and even embarrassing. Men should not have to change their lifestyle to accommodate the symptoms of an enlarged prostate, but they do.

OTHER SOURCES OF PROSTATE ENLARGEMENT

BPH arises from hormonal alterations that are part of aging. Other conditions for prostate enlargement can also block urine flow and some forms may not be benign.

PROSTATITIS is an inflammation of the prostate and may be painful. Prostatitis is common in adult males and falls into four categories:

acute prostatitis
chronic bacterial prostatitis (1.&2. account for 5% of total cases)
Nonbacterial prostatitis comprises 64% of cases.
Prostatodynia accounts for 31% of cases.

SYMPTOMS OF PROSTATE ENLARGEMENT

The inability to empty the bladder happens when the enlarged prostate puts pressure on the urethra. Retained urine can cause nocturia (loss of sleep), inability to control urine flow (incontinence), and retained urine can also cause bacterial growth and infection.

The above sources that encourage prostate enlargement can be painful due to inflammatory conditions. In the case of BPH, there is not an acute form of pain, but it can be uncomfortable.

Acute prostatitis can be found in sexually active men who have a number of sexual partners.

Chronic prostatitis can be related to lack of treatment for acute prostates, or it may develop on its own. It can involve low-level infections and the symptoms include frequent and painful urination as well as sleep interruptions.

Nonbacterial prostatitis is the most common of conditions. Symptoms include post-ejaculatory pain and discomfort. There seems to be no conventional medical treatment (see natural therapies). Lifestyle changes should include elimination of alcohol and spicy foods.

Prostatodynia shares many symptoms of the above conditions, but it lacks high levels of inflammatory cells. Symptoms that are peculiar to prostatodynia, include pain in the groin, perineum, testicles, lower back and penis. Smooth muscle spasms in the prostatic portion of the urethra and in the neck of the bladder are present.

AMERICAN UROLOGICAL ASSOCIATION SYMPTOM INDEX

For questions 1-6, score 0 for not at all; 1 for less than 1 time in 5; 2 for less than ½ the time; 3 for about ½ the time; 4 for more than half the time; 5 for almost always. YOUR SCORE (0,1,2,3,4 OR 5)

Over the past month or so, how often have you had a feeling of not emptying your bladder completely after you finishing urination?

Over the past month or so, how often have you had to urinate again less than two hours after you finished urinating?

Over the past month or so, how often have you found you stopped and started again several times when you urinated?

Over the past month or so, how often have you found it difficult to postpone urination?

Over the past month or so, how often have you had a weak urinary stream?

Over the past month or so, how often have you had to push or strain to begin urinating?

Over the last month, how many times did you most typically get up to urinate from the time you went to bed at night until the time you got up in the morning? (0,1,2,3,4, or 5)

SCORING.

The sums of the answer scores give us the severity of the BPH as follows:

0-7 = mild prostatism

8-18 = moderate prostatism

19-35 = severe prostatism

HORMONES AND THE PROSTATE

Male Menopause?

While there is acceptance about the changing ratios of testosterone and estrogen in both men and women during the aging process, there is little understanding why the ratio and clearance changes in men lead to the enlargement of the prostate. Women have increases in testosterone, while men have a rise in estrogen levels.

Testosterone, the male hormone, peaks during adolescence, and then begins to decrease. Around the age of 50, the sharp decline in testosterone fosters the development of DHT (5-alpha-dihydrotestosterone). Testosterone is converted to DHT by an enzyme called 5-alpha-reductase. The action of DHT is believed to cause the enlargement of the prostate. DHT binds to specific receptors on prostate cells, the alpha 1-receptors. It is then transported to the nucleus of the prostate cells where it attaches to the DNA and turns on prostate growth.

Both drugs and botanical products have been found to ameliorate enlarged prostate conditions.

TREATMENT FOR BPH AND PROSTATITIS

The lack of information related to the treatment of BPH and prostatitis might lead some men to a physician's office and, too often, low levels of problems related to enlarged prostates are treated with drugs.

It is critical to visit a physician's office when the symptoms become acute. Men might exacerbate their conditions when they use only natural products, so the decision should be based on the types and level of symptoms.

DRUG therapies include the following pharmaceuticals: PROSCAR, HYTRIN AND FLOMAX. Proscar has been in the news recently and the results have been mixed. Proscar is also referred to as finasteride. This drug is moderately successful in reducing the size of the prostate, and also ameliorating some of the urinary symptoms associated with BPH. Unfortunately, it takes as long as six months before it becomes effective.

According to the Norris Cancer Institute of the University of California study, the risk of certain prostate cancers is increased dramatically when Proscar is used.

The side effects include decreased libido, premature ejaculation and impotence. Another negative feature has to do with exposure to women who are pregnant. Contact with this drug can cause birth defects. Another problem is the fact that it elevates the PSA (prostate-specific antigen) score up to 60%.

HYTRIN AND FLOMAX are another class of drugs called alpha-blockers. They act by relaxing the smooth muscle of the prostate gland and the neck of the bladder which help improve urine flow.

Side effects include headaches, fatigue, nasal congestion, dizziness and sudden unconsciousness. This class of drugs are usually temporary and the prostate continues to enlarge and then surgery may be necessary.

NATURAL REMEDIES play an important role in the treatment of prostate problems. In Europe, botanicals are approved by a process that insures the product is consistent in its activity and molecular makeup. Products in the approved monograph class include saw palmetto, nettle, and pygeum. Another product that is relatively obscure in the USA is flower pollen extract.

The medical community needs to be more educated to prostate problems that can be solved by natural products that have no side effects. Too often many of the problems do not need drug therapy and it is necessary for people to recognize where they stand in regards to treatment.

Saw Palmetto is perhaps the most well known natural remedy for BPH. It can inhibit the enzyme 5-alpha reductase and this results in a lower production of DHT. The internet can be an excellent source of information on this sybject, such as the Physician's Desk Reference (PDR) for Nutritional Supplements (located on Amazon.com). This is well written and authoritative, and includes research data either supporting claims or disputing them. It is important to deal with brands of products that have the blessing of the physician that you have selected to handle your specific prostate problem.

Rye Pollen Extracts (Prexamed), has a wider scope of activity. It acts as an anti-inflammatory, smoothing muscles involved in urination, stopping the creation of, and the bleeding to, prostate cells of DHT. Head to head studies have revealed it has more benefits than other phyto-pharmaceutical remedies, and can work in one to three months.

Another entry into the mix is the extraction of a molecule called Beta-Sitosterol. This approach seems to have caught on and the entire botanical line of remedies has grown, especially due to the safety they possess.

The key to buying products might be as simple as "it works for me." It is important to realize that the studies utilize certain formulations and other similar products do not qualify for use of this information. Science is now involved in the creation, testing and development of these new natural medicines, and it is vital to know that all the products are not the same. Too often the manufacturers purchase sub par materials and this can lead to poor quality and a lack of potency on the label. Buyer beware!

A good source of information is found in the PDR for Nutritional Supplements. This is well written and authoritative, and includes research data either supporting claims or disputing them.

Chapter 19

ONE MAN'S BURNING, BUT BENIGN, PROGRESS WITH HIS PROSTATE

Don Regan

A Greenhorn at Age 58

This saga springs from one significant sized (large apricot) prostate which lay dormant for 57 years. Then it led its owner on a jarring urinary journey during the otherwise tranquil autumn of life.

Not uncommonly, the onset occurred without warning. Late one night, at a farm B&B in the middle of Maine, my prostate and I attended the rehearsal dinner prior to the wedding of my best friend's daughter. The groom and groomsmen were a hardy bunch of Maine forest rangers who naturally tapped a keg to steel the groom for the upcoming nuptials. Defending the honor of California beach boys, I went mug for mug with these lads. No problem …until about midnight when, back at the farm, I got up to take a leak and couldn't turn the faucet on. As pain began to replace surprise, the power grid for the entire central Maine went out, so there were no communications from or lights in the isolated farmhouse. The total population of this large sector of central Maine was just slightly over 1000, scattered through small villages imaginatively and internationally named (Sweden, Norway, France). After a two hour drive guided only by the rental car's headlights, we finally located a small hospital north of Norway. I rushed in but not quite quickly enough. Five minutes previously the victims of a major automobile accident had been delivered to the ER and the entire staff was in triage mode serving those whose injuries (but not pain) were worse. After about 1½ hours of doing the squirm dance in, around and throughout the hospital, an angel from heaven (aka nurse) arrived with a catheter. Those readers who have experienced the intensity and helplessness resulting from several hours of blockage, followed by the immediate ecstasy of unplugging, know the feeling.

Then followed a brand new, but eventually all too familiar ritual: catheter in; fluid out; bag taped to thigh (right hang). So equipped, I was able to attend the wedding, toast in champagne, even dance a waltz, and, so long as fully clothed, lead a normal looking life. We celebrated Maine in the summer, which was August 7th that year.

After removing the plug and a couple of days of rest, it appeared the problem was solved. Unfortunately, it was just chapter one of the painful hegira. A leisurely drive to Boston led directly to two seats in row one of a 747 headed to LAX. As we sipped our champagne and the plane backed away from the gate, the seizure hit again. Staying calm I asked the stewardess if she were a nurse and had a catheter aboard. Otherwise I couldn't make the 6+ hour flight. She quickly conferred with the pilot who, fortunately, was a member of the ubiquitous brotherhood of the previously plugged. With educated empathy, he taxied back to the gate and deposited my wife and me, carrying only a briefcase and handbag, for transportation to Boston General. The way to the awaiting crisis solving catheter, as those familiar with Boston know only too well, goes through the continuously clogged Callanan tunnel. During the 40 minutes it took us to inch into town, the tunnel wasn't the only thing that was clogged. Once at Boston General, however, relief was almost immediate. The implementing intern was a young man from Balboa who, fortunately for me, chose Harvard medical over Harvard law to pursue his studies. I rewarded him with a sloppy, heartfelt kiss (of the Russian military, not the San Francisco marrying variety).

Equipped with catheter and bag, I returned to California just in time to suit up for a World Senior Games qualifying volleyball tournament as part of the California Beach Boys, of whom Mike O'Hara, this tome's author, was a teammate. Uniformed in baggy sweatpants, I played the full tournament (adequately I assume – ask Mike), which we won and qualified for the World Games.

Nevertheless, since sweatpants prevented display of manly legs on the beach, a more lasting fix was required.

Laser Surgery – Treatment #1

At that time I was a director of a company which manufactured lithotripters and dealt extensively with urologists throughout the world. Our chairman researched the field and came up with what he said were two of the best in California. I chose Jeffrey Kaufman, MD, who checked me out and scheduled a procedure at 9 am at the Western Medical Center. He told me I would be out of the hospital on the same day, would have a few weeks rehab, during which time I could not work out. So, when I arrived at the hospital at 7 am, I thought it would be prudent to do three laps up and down six floors of stairs prior to the procedure. To those with a better understanding of physiology than I, after the uneventful laser procedure, my blood still pumped at intensified levels and earned me an extra night and day in the hospital.

On discharge I was given a short lecture and an explanation of how the Laser had taken the rough edges off the insides of my oversize prostate, with the hope for a long term (several years) respite from the stoppage problem. Most comfortingly, all studies showed that I was only a minor victim –BPH, no malignancy.

Microwave – Round #2

For a few years, no problems. Then one fine day I was making a presentation to the city council in the town of San Bernardino, about 55 miles from Dr. Kaufman's office. In mid sentence the malady struck again. The pain was immediate. While still able to speak coherently, I asked the council for a recess. They said "Sure, how long?" I said "A couple of weeks." "What?" came the chorus. As I explained that my prostate had crept unsuspectingly up on me, the mayor, fortunately another of the previously plugged brethren, raised his hand, said "I understand", and gave me his phone to call Dr.

Kaufman, who generously agreed to stay through lunch to act as an angel of mercy. The mayor provided me with a police escort out of town which dumped me on Interstate 10 West. After a few miles, total gridlock. Up ahead a truck loaded with gravel had tipped over and spread its load across all westbound lanes. I found myself stopped in the right lane, punching the car ceiling with my left hand and pulling on my beleaguered unit with the right. Unfortunately, my neighbor high up on the left was driving an eighteen wheeler. As he looked down at my playful gyrations, he responded with a few knowing winks. Resisting his blandishments, I pulled out onto the shoulder and began speeding through the gravel towards Dr. Kaufman's waiting fingers. Uh-oh, just as I was emerging ahead of the pack, a CHP officer blocked my path. Again, my gutsy guardian angel, obviously not yet fatigued, glided to my rescue. I rolled down the window to explain my plight. It fell on instantly empathetic ears, for the officer was a member in good standing of the Blocked Brotherhood. He not only waved me through, but radioed ahead so that I got a pat on the rear as I sped west. Dr. Kaufman again caressed me with the catheter and scheduled another procedure.

A few days later, this time totally relaxed, I was again at Western Med and the procedure, as it was explained to me, resembled a microwave lawnmower mowing down the stalagmites and stalactites which remained after the Laser procedure. After a short rehab, again back to normal life – no problem, but not permanent.

Slice & Dice – the third and final(?) chapter

Several years later and back on the beach in Irvine Cove was the scene for another rehearsal dinner hosted by an Irish cousin. Again it was necessary to have a jar or two to show eastern members of the Regan/Murphy/Welch sect that west coasters are not effete. As the stars came out, the band played Four Green Fields and other rebel songs to which we clansmen spun off a jig and a few reels.

The first problem sign occurred when I went to the gents to shake the mayor's hand and pass the night's beer through my urinary tract: several drops of blood accompanied the stream.

Less than an hour later, the familiar pain, only more intense, began and the flow of blood increased and led straight to the emergency room at Hoag Hospital in Newport Beach. After the now customary catheter, study of my prostate by the urologist on duty showed lesions which had parted giving rise to the unwanted red river. Suggestion, even with the attendant risks: this time allow the knife to scrape the interior wall. I said OK to this serious surgery. Surgery succeeded, but recovery required hooking me up to hydrate water in and let blood and urine out. Consequently, I spent two days attached to more tubes than an octopus has arms. Recuperation, however, produced enduring memories:

The strong post operative recommendation was that, for anticipated nocturnal pain, I take a serious pain killer, i.e. Demoral. Having experienced the Elysian Fields of fantasy courtesy of Demoral during recuperation from an adult tonsillectomy, I said no and was determined to gut it out. Along about 3 am, however, the pain won and I buzzed for the nurse. When she arrived, she started laughing and informed me of the traditional good news, bad news scenario:

The bad news was that I was in real pain and needed the painkiller immediately;

The good news, delivered before a growing audience, was that my ability to perform manly marital maneuvers was no longer in question – the pain was caused by a gigantic erection which dislodged the tube running through the interior of my tattered but true talisman.

Next day, three of my Welch cousins, all experienced prostaters, while on their way home from the wedding to Iowa, paid a palliative visit. Being thoughtful and Irish they brought a generous goodwill memento. Their get well creation consisted of two large black ball shaped balloons tied stoutly but suggestively to the base of a long thin white balloon, the tip of which was a poignant recovery note. Naturally, on the way in, the three Welches danced with each and every nurse on the entire floor and were prevented only by an early curfew from turning an otherwise sedate surgery ward into a Dublin Pub.

This send off must be largely responsible for the fact that since leaving Hoag, I have been able to whiz like a teenager, have had no blood, and have been able to fulfill responsibilities, in spite of the minor inconvenience known as retrograde ejaculation, in the best tradition of a 69 year old practicing monogamist in frequent pursuit of his bride of 48 years who helped live through and laugh at this voyage through unabridged, but benign urinary territories.

CONCLUSION AND THE FUTURE

The compelling conclusion is that I am indeed fortunate to be benign. Nevertheless, in my case, the laser and microwave attempts to avoid the knife proved to be temporary solutions to impeding the relentless growth of the prostate. Thus, while all three technologies work, "slice and dice" even with its anticipated side effects provided the more complete conclusion.

Next, based on my experience as a knowledgeable medical consumer and the salvation and longevity of the many men I have referred to him, Jeffrey Kaufman must be a Pro's Pro.

Lessons learned by which to shape present and future conduct include:

Hydrate (10+ glasses of water daily), even though this increases the WD-40 budget to make sure the constant fly unzipping goes as smoothly as possible.

Relax (breathe deeply, let the jaw go slack), exercise vigorously and sleep lots (a prophylactic prescription).

Continuing blood tests and exams (learn to love, not fear, your friendly physician's middle digit).

Keep the PMA (Positive Medical Attitude) high and the PSA low.

Don't bother with Saw Palmetto, beta blockers and other feel-good formulae – practice #2 above and leave the supplements to Barry Bonds.

As a result of these items 1-5 plus good luck, today my body resembles an old balsa wood surfboard, sturdy, but with many splinters split and gone. The board (body) still floats and can be paddled out to enjoy the surf, so I continue to catch, with gusto, the waves of life.

Don Regan
Age 69
Balboa, CA

Chapter 20

OBSERVATIONS REGARDING RADICAL PROSTATE SURGERY

by Richard Archer

Having now experienced radical prostate surgery I expect others contemplating the surgery will likewise contact me to get non-medical views on the surgical procedure. As such, I want to reduce to writing these non-medical observations so that hopefully I can be helpful to those who inquire. I've found the information available from physicians on prostate surgery is better than that which I could locate regarding my previous surgeries.

My initial "impression" of radical prostate surgery was that this procedure was pretty routine. After all "the prostate is only the size of a walnut or apricot and was no big deal - kind of like cutting off an ingrown cyst." WRONG! This is major surgery and requires great skill by the surgeon and his operating team. On the spot judgments must be made by the surgeon during roughly a 2-1/2 hour procedure.

I was very surprised at the length of time required to recover from surgery. This was largely because of my mistaken "impression" since I totally underestimated the severity of the surgery and how much physically, along with the general anesthetic, this took out of you. I was told after the surgery that I was doing very well but since I had no comparative standard I had no way to evaluate those observations. In retrospect, seven weeks after the surgery I think I probably did quite well.

Also I recognize that each patient is unique and different. While there are many similarities there are many differences. What works for one person won't necessarily work for another. With those reservations stated above, I offer the following comments:

Selection of Surgeon. This is a very difficult and strangely emotional exercise, but in my view necessary in order to assure yourself of the most expert of care. In my situation I started with a urologist recommended by my internist who I believe was adequately qualified. However, I did obtain recommendations from other people when they learned of my condition, and after receiving a second opinion I did select Dr. Jean deKernion who is the Chief of Division of Urology at the UCLA School of Medicine. As it turns out I am pleased that I made this selection, but of course that is not to imply (since I will never know) that the first surgeon might not also have performed a successful surgery.

The only thing that I can say when checking around with people whose options I highly regard is that I find two names in the Southern California area tend to surface more than any other: Dr. Don Skinner - Kenneth Norris Cancer Clinic USC School of Medicine and Dr. Jean deKernion - UCLA School of Medicine.

The point I want to make here is that you should check around with people you respect and then make a decision. I would also caution against "falling in love with your physician" since that is usually the case when someone has realized a successful surgery.

Procedures Needed Prior to Surgery. It is necessary to check with your insurance company regarding admission to a hospital. Most of them don't like your going in the night before since it costs an extra day. If that is the case and it is necessary to check into the hospital at, say, 7:00 a.m., it is best for you to schedule your surgery at 11:00 a.m. or later in that day if that is a viable option.

You will want to store up two or three units (1 pint each) of your own blood and this is best done at the hospital in which the surgery will be performed. This is referred to as autologous blood donations and you can do this approximately one week apart. You will be given iron pills to build up your iron count and also vitamin C which should be taken as prescribed between times when you give blood.

You will need a CAT Scan as well as a Bone Scan, preferably at the hospital where surgery is performed. My impression is that the CAT Scan is isolated in the pelvic area to identify, for the surgeon, needed information regarding organs surrounding the prostate. A Bone Scan, as I understand it, is to determine whether any malignancy has shown up in any of your bone structure. Collectively these procedures involve two-thirds of the day since part of it involves nuclear medicine and requires shots at certain intervals for the test to be properly read.

Preparation Prior To Entering The Hospital. A special diet requires usually clear liquids for two days prior to surgery and also necessary bowel preparation one day prior to the surgery. Regarding the Citrate of Magnesia, which really is a laxative, I would suggest that you chill that prior to taking it since it tends to kill the taste and is more palatable. Other than that, the enemas specified are pretty standard procedure. However, despite all this I was still required to take a medicated enema the morning of surgery.

Shaving all bodily hair, including all pubic hair, is a must. I would suggest that one shave themselves clear of hair on the front side of their body from 2" above the belly button to 2" below the pelvis, which of course, would include both legs. The surgeon does not want hair to get in the way and believe me, you do not want it present in areas where adhesive tape will be applied.

One might consider shaving their lower arms maybe half way up the elbow since you will have a number of IV's which are taped and blood tests which after being taken also involve tape. That should be strictly optional and I did not choose to do it. As regards shaving around genital areas clearly someone needs to be careful. Actually, the nurse did that on me since we were short of time when I entered the hospital. That job is not as easy to do by you, the individual involved, as you might think.

Timing of Hospital Admission. I've alluded to this earlier under the pre-op section. It is probably important to recognize that if you check into the hospital the day of your surgery, delaying the surgery until later is probably a good idea. After the surgery I was given Heparin which is a blood thinner, the purpose of which is to avoid blood clots. I had to delay using the pain machine, because of the Heparin. I'm told that I would have been given the shot earlier (1-2 hours before surgery) had I entered the hospital the night before. I was informed that many surgeons don't believe in using Heparin.

Surgical Room. Things go pretty rapidly when you are delivered to surgery, so be prepared for a room with a lot of bright lights and a high level of activity. You certainly will be able to get up on the surgical table yourself, but you will shortly not be conscious as the general anesthesia is administered soon after you arrive.

Day of Surgery. As mentioned earlier, you will have been shaved either by yourself prior to admission or by a nurse at the hospital. Also, they will provide you with a medicated enema in all probability. In my own experience, the anesthetist also visited me to determine if I was allergic to any drugs, etc. Also, the surgeon will visit to explain the last minute procedures and to get various releases permitting him to do certain things within the surgery that may be necessary on the spot.

Post Operative - In Hospital Equipment. There are four things that will be standard equipment. The first is known as a pain machine which is hooked into the IV line and allows for dispensing of pain killing medicine (morphine) on a controlled basis. This is really only needed for the two or three days following surgery but is helpful. Also, there is now a pump to inflate a bladder type device that is wrapped around each leg in order to stimulate leg blood circulation. This, among other things, presumably tends to avoid blood clots and keeps the blood circulating. The IV is standard procedure as this is the way you will get your nourishment for three to four days including various antibiotics. The other item is the catheter bag into which the urine will flow from the catheter tube which is attached to you.

Post Operative Surgical Exterior Physical Result. The location of the incision is approximately from the bottom of the belly button to about 1" above the penis. This involves an incision approximately 5" long. There is another incision about 1-1/2" on diagonal used for a drain to which a bandage is applied to allow for and soak up whatever drainage there might be. On me, this was on the left side about 4" below the belly button and on a diagonal. The center incision will be closed by staples and those staples will be removed generally at the time you leave the hospital.

Exercise in Hospital. The only exercise you actually get will be walking and usually you will be taken out of bed the second day after surgery. There is some pain in first getting out of bed, but certainly tolerable. I was surprised that it is quite an effort merely to walk ten feet. Don't let that concern you as your walking will increase geometrically each day. You will find that you can walk in the hospital corridors and even attach your catheter urine bag and the pain machine to a pole on casters that you can roll with you. It sounds a little bizarre but everybody else does it so don't let it concern you. I found by the fourth day that I could walk the full hallway of the hospital wing in which I was located and I believe walking is helpful and very important as it tends to get your system moving. Also, you will be encouraged to move your feet and legs while in bed to minimize the risk of clotting in the legs.

IV. As mentioned earlier, you will be fed by an IV and normally you can expect to be on that for the day of surgery plus the three following days. However, I became nauseous on food and because of that was put back on the IV for an additional two days. I am told that is very unusual and could have been caused by the medications. Also,

I started into food that was too rich, too soon. When one starts on a food diet it should be as plain and simple food as possible.

Catheter. The catheter is inserted at the time of surgery so when you actually become conscious it is already installed. The line is taped heavily to your right thigh, approximately 3" from the end of the penis so it will not be moved if the line catches on something. It is important to keep that line clean, especially where the tube enters the penis. Removal of the catheter is quite simple and done by the physician without any pain or problem.

The bag into which the urine flows in the hospital is a pretty big bag and the nurse changes it at needed intervals. The bags that you take home are smaller but quite easy to operate and are good for five days at which time they should be disposed of and a new one used. There is also a small bag that can be attached to the thigh which is handy if you go out in public.

It is possible for you to have what is known as bladder spasm which results in traveling between the catheter tube and the normal and reconnected urinary tract. The result is that it seems like there is a leak and you will get slightly damp. It is no problem but helpful to be aware it can happen.

Also, I had blood congeal in the catheter tube which plugged it up. This built up pressure in the bladder and I (like a bladder spasm) had leakage. This was easily fixed by the nurse who used some sort of syringe to clean out the tube.

Ted Socks. These are what would amount to heavy gauge hose type socks which are placed on both legs to prevent blood clots. You will wear those probably twenty out of the twenty-four hours each day in the hospital. You will need to check with the physician whether you will be required to wear those at home.

Heel Protectors. Your heels tend to get sore when you lay on your back and there are heel protectors which tend to alleviate a soreness somewhat like a blister. You merely need to request these if you have this problem. I think it is the Ted Socks material that irritates the heel and the heel protectors thus are a good idea.

Post Catheter and Bladder Control. There are exercises regarding the bladder that you should follow to strengthen the external sphincter muscle which when developed will now take over and control the flow or urine.

I don't remember the last time I was in diapers, but when the catheter is removed, this becomes necessary. The product I used was called "Depends" which is a line of so called absorbent products. The model known as heavy/complete is for maximum absorbency and probably should be used for the first week after the catheter is removed. Probably it is worth using for three weeks during the night, as when you are sleeping you want this type of protection. After the first week the so called moderate model which involves less bulky material is very satisfactory during the day. After three weeks that should be adequate at night and you will probably use those for about four to five weeks after removal of the catheter. From then on Depends made what they called Shields which are lighter material and can be inserted within a jockey short garment. That really should be adequate after six weeks, at least it was for me.

Bowel Movements. I must say that I never thought the major event for the day would be a bowel movement. It certainly is to the hospital. It is really important to take stool softeners since the internal stitching, with straining, could break loose stitches and become a problem. The important point here is to avoid straining and therefore regular bowel movements and stool softeners are absolutely necessary. I have always been amazed that architects design toilets way too low, especially for tall men and men with long legs. If you only have low toilets at home then it wouldn't be a bad idea to obtain an elevated toilet seat since that tends to avoid strain which otherwise is inherent by the use of a low toilet. Remember that enemas are taboo for a few weeks after surgery.

Lifting and Straining. Your surgeon simply does not want you to lift or strain anything as apparently a lot of organs have been moved around and internal stitching can be damaged. Also, apparently there is concern that you can develop a hernia and this would be quite serious were that repair necessary during your post operative recovery. Certainly, for four weeks after the surgery you should avoid lifting anything that exceeds five pounds. After that you want to be very careful and I would say avoid lifting objects exceeding twenty pounds until probably at least seven to eight weeks after surgery. Again, much of this is individual and you must listen to your physician. At the same point, don't be stupid and create a problem for yourself by lifting or straining.

Approximately two months after my surgery I developed pain in my right leg and believed it was a hip problem. In reality it was a lateral herniated disc in the nerve anal L5 S1. This, believe me, I didn't need. I don't know whether it came from playing golf or my universal exercise machine. What I now realize is your abdominal muscles are wiped out from the prostate surgery. These muscles are important and when firm, strong and developed tend to help carry your spine and back and reduce susceptibility to back strain or damage. I did not apparently allow enough time after surgery before I engaged in exercising. Determine from your surgeon or a therapist how to strengthen the abdominal muscles and ONLY AFTER HEALING IS COMPLETE. I now do a minimum of twenty minutes of stretching and back exercises four days per week to get rid of the back pain. DON'T FORGET THE ADMONITION UNLESS YOU WANT TO DO THIS TWENTY MINUTES A DAY OR WORSE, HAVE THE NEED TO OPT FOR BACK SURGERY.

Erections. You might think it is inappropriate to discuss this here, but at this stage of my life nothing is sacrosanct. On top of that almost every man has asked me about this, so here goes. Apparently there are two nerves on either side of the prostate which are critical in achieving an erection. The surgeon will attempt to save one of the two unless he is concerned the cancer may have attacked it. I am told one of the two nerves is sufficient to achieve an erection. Dr. deKernion was able to save one of the two on me but it hasn't worked. Don't despair. Osbon Medical System has developed a vacuum pump device known as ErecAid System which when used will do the trick. This must be prescribed by your urologist and it is unlikely he will agree until four to six months after surgery. The address is Osbon Medical Systems, 1233 Broad Street, August, GA 30903-1478. Their telephone is 800 346-7266, fax is 706 821-6928. I have not tried it but other male friends who also have had radical prostate surgery tell me you can also take a shot which apparently is very effective. My physician doesn't like the idea because it is invasive. If I insisted he would give me the prescription for the syringe and shot. This is self administered.

Continence. I am fortunate and am at a point where I have full control of my bladder function. This is not the case with some I talk with. However, I find it interesting that those who have taken seriously the exercise for the spincter muscle tend to gain greater control and sooner.

MEMORANDUMS
RICHARD A. ARCHER

Date: November 30, 1995

On Wednesday I had a bone scan at UCLA followed by a pelvic x-ray. While the technician did not tell me, I believe the only reason for the x-ray was because of what he observed in the Bone Scan.

I am scheduled for a CT Scan, 9 a.m., Tuesday, December 5, at UCLA followed by a Needle Biopsy in the prostate area the same day, at 11:45 a.m. This will be done by Dr. Anup Patel, MD I have the antibiotic prescription to be taken before and after the procedure and recognize that a Fleet enema also is required. Dr. Darol Joseff thinks, based on my normal platelet count, that it is OK to proceed.

I am now trying to think ahead recognizing that to wait for each test delays further ultimate treatment for what I now suspect is about a 90% probability. I realize that results of the bone scan and CT scan are needed to establish if cancer is limited to the prostate.

Date: December 13, 1995

With the high probabilities that the malignancy is limited, Dr. deKernion advised me of possible treatments. One would be by the use of hormones which, while it would not kill the cancer, in all probability would control it. The other would be by radiation which, if the cancer is limited to the groin area, would in all probability kill it off. However, before any decision was made on the method of treatment, he wanted me to talk to the Oncologist.

Further, he is specifically concerned that my platelet count has dropped from over 200,000 in April of 1992 to 79,000 today. It is his opinion that a Hematologist must do a needle biopsy of my bone marrow to determine what is going on in this area. He feels this should be done in Santa Barbara. It is important to do this as apparently radiation treatment will sap some of the platelets.

I then met with Dr. Robert Parker who is the radiation oncologist. His view is that the cancer is definitely curable. Further, he states that the radiation will only work if it is applied namely to the pelvic area. He feels I will need the treatment using a Linear Accelerator Radiation Machine. He believes this treatment would be intensive involving seven weeks with five treatments per week. This treatment might be "enhanced" or supplemented by use of pellets. One of the possible side affects of this treatment could be some irritation of the bladder, which can be treated. The other would be soreness of the bowel.

Date: December 20, 1995

First of all of the mystery of the platelet has been solved. Instead of my platelet count being 75,000 it is actually 300,000. I visited Dr. Frederick Kass at the Santa Barbara Hematology Oncology Medical

Group on Tuesday, December 19th, who spent time consulting with me on this issue. He correctly surmised that my platelet bunched and as such, unless you took blood quickly after its being drawn and run the test, it would fall off in count within an hour. He had another patient like this several weeks ago with the same condition. Obviously, whenever blood was drawn in a physician office or lab and then sent out for analysis enough time transpired so the count dropped and thus yeilded an incorrect reading. At least this is behind me and is no problem as respects radiation treatment.

On Wednesday, I consulted with Dr. Thomas Weisenburger at the Radiation Center Medical Group of the Cancer Foundation of Santa Barbara for evaluation of me and alternative treatments. All my records from tests at UCLA were received so he had the benefit of that information. As an alternative (but not substitution) for radiation he felt I should first consider "Androgen Suppression Treatment". This involves one shot per month for three months and the taking of pills four times each day. The purpose of this is to eliminate the affect of testosterone which causes the cancer. Also, it will shrink the cancer in the nodule which everyone has already identified. He does not feel there will be any significant side affects although I may suffer some fatigue. He wished to consult with Dr. Jean deKernion and Dr. Robert Parker, both at UCLA, before deciding on this course. Following consulting with both of them he recommends that I proceed with this treatment prior to any follow-on radiation which he recommends. This will be done by Dr. Frederick Kass.

In about three months, once this is completed, I will undergo radiation treatment. This involves seven weeks with radiation five times per week. Each treatment takes about forty-five minutes from the time you arrive until you leave. Prior to radiation treatment being commenced it will be necessary to have dye injected into the bladder and rectum in order to do a front, side and rear x-ray. The purpose of this is to locate exactly the area to be treated by radiation. Once the treatment is started it is reasonable to assume that the bowel will be affected with the result of some diarrhea. Also, the rectum will be sore and there will be some bladder irritation. Some people become fatigued.

As a rough schedule it would appear that I will commence the Androgen Suppression Treatment the last week of December. Based on this I would start the radiation treatment around April 1, 1996. This will be supervised and monitored by Dr. Weisenburger. Allowing for seven weeks treatment that should be over May 18, 1996.

As I have stated in other memos, I am impressed with the high level of competency of all the physicians I have visited. Out of all this activity of the last six to eight weeks, I think I now comprehend and know what to expect over the next four months.

I have written this memo which hopefully I can use to inform people who need to know of the treatment and schedule that I must follow. Hopefully I can work my other activities around these treatments.

Date: December 28, 1995

On Tuesday, December 26th, I met with Dr. Frederick Kass to learn more regarding the Androgen Suppression Treatment. The net of this is that I will be undergoing this treatment for three months. It involves one shot per month and the taking of one Casodex pill per day. (Dr. Kass will be getting to me regarding more detail and cost this week) Apparently the shot, which I believe is a hormone, virtually shuts off the testosterone in my system and since the prostate cancer cells need testosterone to survive, those cells will die. That should eliminate about 95% of the cells. The Adrenal Gland also generates some cells and the pills are designed to zap those cells. Dr. Kass was careful and thorough to explain to me that the use of pills is not mandatory but he highly recommends using them. The reason is this treatment is still undergoing evaluation but the results to date have been very favorable. The pills are expensive and he brought this to my attention. The bottom line on this treatment is that it will shrink the tumor and temporarily kill off the cells. However, radiation following will finish them off for good. I got the first shot on December 26th and there is no noticeable side affects. I will have full flexibility during these three months as respects activity and movement. I have scheduled the second shot for Thursday, January 25, 1996 and the third shot for Friday, February 23, 1996.

As mentioned in my memo of December 20, 1995, I will start the radiation treatment at the Santa Barbara Radiation Center Medical Group of the Cancer Foundation of Santa Barbara on Monday, April 1, 1996. This involves one treatment per day for five days per week for seven weeks. This will hold me close to home except for some round trips to Los Angeles. The expected side affects will be some irritation of the bowl, rectum and bladder. Also, it is reasonable to expect some diarrhea as well as experience some fatigue. All of this is controllable.

Hopefully, after all of this the cancer will be eliminated and I can schedule out the next forty years of my life!

Date: June 7, 1996

I have now completed five full months of treatment using Lupron and Casodex as well as radiation involving thirty-eight treatments five times per week for seven and one half weeks. It has been an interesting and challenging time. I want to record some of my impressions which hopefully will be helpful to others who will undergo this same treatment.

The Androgen Suppression Treatment is pretty straight forward. I had a Lupron shot once per month and at this point have had five shots. Also, I take one Casodex pill per day. The only reaction seems to be occasional "hot flashes." Other than that I noticed no additional side affects. It seems to have worked as suggested as after three months my PSA dropped from 9.2 to 0.2. The urologist/oncologist estimated that the tumor in my groin shrunk 75% which gave a smaller area to treat with radiation. Dr. Kass feels current research suggests that I continue this treatment for two months post radiation.

Approximately April 1st I started radiation. The following are my observations in outline topic form:

1. This is a daily routine which in the aggregate takes about one and one half hours per day. Fortunately Cottage Hospital is only fifteen minutes driving from the house. By the time you leave the home, drive to the hospital, change into your hospital gown, wait and get your radiation, get dressed again, and drive home, one and one half hours has elapsed. Since you should not miss any treatments you are confined to this general location. However, I did go to Los Angeles for the day and night as well as to San Francisco.

2. The following are my impressions regarding the effect that this treatment had on me:

    a. The Linear Accelerator (X-ray machine) is a big machine that is rotated around you. I was zapped from three sides taking about fifteen to twenty seconds per zap. (They didn't do the fourth side as my steel prosthesis from the hip replacement blocked access to the area). Actually, you do not feel anything during these treatments.

    b. The first three weeks I felt no fatigue and functioned as I always did. I am told that radiation has a cumulative effect and builds up in your body. After the third week I took about a one hour nap per day. The last two weeks I did notice I would tire more.

    c. As far as physical change in the body the most pronounced was my rectum. After about three weeks I started to get sore and the burn cream didn't do the job. This is known as "Aquaphor" and is a healing ointment. I rubbed it on all external areas where the radiation was applied, after each treatment. Bowel movements were a little painful but nothing serious. The reaction was somewhat like hemorrhoids. The nurse suggested using witch hazel or a commercial product known as Tucks which contains witch hazel. This seemed to relieve the itching. However, eventually apparently the skin cracked in one area so the nurse took me off witch hazel and suggested soaking in the bath tub for twenty to thirty minutes daily. The physician also prescribed Proctosol-HC 2.5% which is Hydrocortisone Cream. I would apply this about four times per day and this worked very well. After thirty-eight treatments my rear end was quite tender. There was no irritation on the side but some minor soreness in the upper penis area. It is important to use the Aquaphor as this area is easily burned.

d. Apparently the radiation hits the lower part of your bladder so you feel the need to urinate more often. Sometimes you have the urge "to go" even though there is very little to discharge. If you wait this urge subsides. As far as bowel movements are concerned all was quite normal and I never experienced diarrhea. I attribute this to good diet and following instructions given at the beginning of treatment regarding prohibited food. During the entire period I maintained a good appetite and lost about five pounds.

3. As mentioned previously I believe diet is of great importance when you undergo this treatment. Fortunately for me Jean was great in preparing the right kind of meals and I religiously followed the instructions on prohibited food. I did cheat by drinking wine but cut back on that. A vegetarian diet and avoiding much in the way of dairy products and red meat is important. Also, to make up I drank a heavy daily dose of "Shaklee's Protein Supplement." That maintained my energy level.

4. The post radiation treatment time has been interesting as two days after my last radiation treatment I was off to Hawaii. The physicians told me it would take ten days before I was fully back

to normal. I really thought it would be sooner. However, now having been thirteen days I found that they were right. I took at least a one hour nap each day and slept long nights. I could feel a healing process within my body where the good cells were being reinstated.

I did not feel like doing too much, and no golf. After nine days I did start playing golf as well as more swimming. Also, the Mai Tais have had a very positive effect!

5. Now with my experience behind me I have asked myself the question "what would I have done differently?" I think preempting the problem with the rectum would have been smart. First of all I would use Baby Wipes (non alcohol) after bowel movements from day one. It was the toilet paper rubbing against very tender skin that eventually ruptured the skin. I would also have done more soaking earlier in the treatment. You must treat your rear end with "ever loving care". Secondly, I took on a project of installing and learning Windows 95 on my new computer. I don't think mentally I was as sharp as usual and I think this added to my fatigue. As such I would not take on anything new but just keep on doing only the essentials.

At this point I will be ready in two more weeks to be examined by the urologist/oncologist to see how the radiation treatment worked. Hopefully it did and time will tell.

As I mentioned at the beginning of this memo, I am recording this with the thought that some of the experiences and observations I had will be helpful to others. This diagnostic process started in September 1995 so it has now been nine months. I would also like to state that I have had absolutely the best of treatment from the physicians, nurses and technicians who have treated me. I owe them all a great deal and am most appreciative of their work. Additionally, the understanding and patience of my wife Jean has been of great help and support.

Date: February 10, 1997

It is now thirteen months since I started the prostate cancer treatment and seven months since my interim report of June 7, 1996. It is apparent that my treatment concerning both the chemo and the radiation therapy were very effective.

I continued the Lupron shots monthly and the taking of Casodex pills daily through the month of August, or eight full months. My PSA is below 0.1 and virtually imperceptible. I am now on a schedule to see Dr. Kass and Dr. Weisenburger at six month intervals. Therefore, I see one every three months. The purpose of this is to monitor my condition and watch for any reoccurrence.

Date: July 5, 2000

Following treatment in 1996-1997 I visited the oncologist every three months and also had a PSA test once per month for monitoring. It held at about 0.01 for approximately two years. Then in early 1998 it climbed to 4.5. At that point Dr. Fred Kass put me back on Luprin and Casodex. The hormonal therapy worked fine and after about one year the PSA was back to 0.01. I continued to have the PSA test monthly and visited Dr. Kass quarterly. In November 1999 the PSA started to climb. In February 2000 Dr. Kass put me back on Zolodex 3.6MG (substitute for Luprin) as the PSA was at 4.5. Three months later the PSA had gone up to 9.0. At this point I was put on Casodex and Proscar. This stabilized the PSA and it has not gone up any further.

I am told if the hormonal treatment does not respond I will then need to pursue a more aggressive therapy (chemotherapy). However, Dr. Kass wants to hold me in this pattern as long as possible since there are many new and better treatments coming on line.

As such, this is an ever continuing saga.

Date: July 5, 2000

When I review all the memos going back to early 1992 I am surprised with how much treatment I had over that period of time.

Throw in a right hip replacement, and it is no wonder that Medi-Care is running out of money. Maybe old volleyball players need new hips and have prostate problems!

I would not want anyone reading these memos to use them for any more than general information. As always, a patient must seek the best physician he can find and then follow his advice. That has not changed. However, prostate cancer treatment has improved significantly especially with the introduction of the needle implants. I have learned that about thirty percent of patients who have radical prostate surgery ultimately have the prostate cancer return. I am in that thirty percent.

Based on what I know today, including the experiences of some of the individuals who will contribute to the book, I would never opt for radical prostate surgery. I say that because the hormonal treatment and needle implants accomplish virtually the same thing without the risk and potential subsequent problems resulting from radical prostate surgery. A number of people have incontinence and penile erection problems as a result of surgery. At least now with the use of Viagra, this helps with penile erection, if you can wait an hour for it to work! I would only undergo radical prostate surgery after obtaining two opinions from urologists other than surgeons.

I simply do not know what the future has in store for me but at age seventy-three I will keep plodding along with the hope that something else will get me before prostate cancer.

Chapter 21

MY PROSTATE CANCER SHOCK

by Jack Schumacher

For my entire life of 68 years I have always been the picture of health. I have never had any major sickness or abnormalities. My life has always been lived in moderation with regular exercise, proper dietary control, little stress, never had high blood pressure, a non-smoker and been very happily married for 38 years.

So I asked myself, how could this happen to me?

It all happened in July 1999 when I applied for some additional life insurance to be added to my estate plan. As we all know life insurance requires a basic insurance physical involving blood, urine specimen, and a resting EKG. The blood results came back with a PSA (Prostate Specific Antigen) reading of 4.5. My insurance company informed me I had crossed over the line of 4.0 for a standard preferred rate, but most important my PSA reading had jumped in one year from 3.2 to 4.5. Hearing the news it alarmed me enough to schedule an immediate complete physical from my internist, which was scheduled two weeks after my insurance exam. To my shock my new PSA reading jumped again, even higher up to 6.7. While this doesn't necessarily mean I have prostate cancer, to play it safe my physician referred me to an urologist for an ultra sound examination and a biopsy of my prostate. I went to see Dr. Mark Kelly who performed this procedure and then sent the report off to a pathology lab in Oklahoma City for evaluation. Four days later, Dr. Kelly called me and said, "I don't know how to tell you this, but you have prostate cancer". At first hearing this news, I was totally devastated. How could this happen to me, I asked myself. I am a physically fit 68 year old male, don't smoke, drink very little, eat the right health foods, no cancer history in my family, so how could this happen to me? It took me two or three days to emotionally adjust to my medical problem.

Like most men I was basically uninformed about prostate cancer. The first thing my internist suggested I do was find a bookstore and buy Dr. Patrick C. Walsh's (Director of the Department of Urology at John Hopkins University School of Medicine) book titled "The Prostate - a Guide for Men and the Women who love them." I bought the book and immediately read all 400 pages.

My next move was to telephone some of my close friends whom I knew had encountered this same problem over the past 6 years to see if they could provide me with their input as to what direction I should take. I learned there are various treatments you can take, none of which are totally full proof. Each man has to make his own decision based on his comfort zone. The different options are as follows:

Radical Prostatectomy - surgical removal
Nerve Sparing Prostatectomy - surgical removal saving bundle nerves
External Beam Radiation - exterior radiation over 7 weeks
"Seed" Radiation - implant radiation
Cryotherapy - freezing of prostate
Hormone Therapy - loss of libido - cancer may return within a few years
Do Nothing - hoping for a new cure drug to come on the market in the near future

In order to decide which way I should proceed I needed to know the severity of my prostate cancer. From the pathology report my prostate was diagnosed okay on the left side with a Mid Gleason 6 (3+3) but on the right side, my right base was a Gleason 7 (3+4) and the right mid Gleason 7 (3+4). I was told my cancer was in the very beginning stages and probably had not gone through the capsule.

I was advised by my physician to get a second and third opinion and seek out the most skilled and experienced urologist surgeons. So I scheduled an appointment to meet with Dr. Robert B. Smith at the Clark Urology Institute at UCLA School of Medicine and with Dr. Donald Skinner at the Kenneth Norris Cancer Clinic USC School of Medicine. I felt it important to see these physicians since they are involved with teaching hospitals and are dealing more with state of the art surgery through their continuous research.

Seven out of the ten friends I contacted opted for the Nerve Sparing Prostatectomy procedure and two because of their ages (over 75) elected for the external beam radiation and one decided to do nothing. He was the youngest, age 56. He felt a new therapeutic strategy might be available in the not to distance future, called E-Catherine Protein, which stops the release of enzymes known to play a role in cancer invasion, perhaps this will happen, I hope so for his sake. Personally though, I would not want to risk waiting, particularly if you are dealing with cancer.

Since my prostate cancer was just in the very beginning stages, I felt the Radical Prostatectomy surgery was the safest approach.

When I met with Dr. Donald Skinner for the first time, it became very easy for me to select him to do my surgery. He is head of cancer research at USC Norris Cancer Center with an impeccable reputation. It is very important to get two or three opinions and it is very important to select a physician who has done this surgery many times. Some questions you must ask the surgeon are as follows:

How many prostate operations do you do a year?
What success have you had in preserving potency and continence?
Have you done at least 400 surgeries?

Dr. Skinner answered all of these questions to my total satisfaction.

He said your chances are excellent. With regard to still being continent after the surgery, he said he has had a 98% success rate over the years. After hearing this, I said lets go with it! I had two out of town trips I planned to take during the next month, I told Dr. Skinner I would scrub both of them and come in next week, if you can schedule me. He said no - take your trips, in the meantime, I will prescribe a female hormone pill for you to take twice a day for 7 weeks prior to the surgery and then we will operate.

Regarding the surgery, I had read where surgical blood transfusions would be required. Dr. Skinner said: "No, we have a safe blood bank here at the Norris Cancer Center but it's a rarity we ever need to give a blood transfusion. Four or five years earlier it was necessary. Today because of new surgery techniques the vast majority of our patients will not require a transfusion". I wanted to know how long the surgery would take. I was told approximately 1 1/2 hours. Dr. Skinner pointed out because he prescribed the female hormone pills the prostate would shrink somewhat making it easier for surgical removal. I made it clear to Dr. Skinner I hoped he would be able to spare my bundle nerves on both sides. He said there is a 90% chance he would be successful because my cancer was just in the beginning stages.

My surgery was performed at 7:30 am, September 27, 1999 and took approximately one hour and 28 minutes. I was out of recovery at 10:30 am and later that afternoon I was out of bed taking my first steps. The next day I was walking the halls. Since my post operative condition was a non-event and I was encountering little or no pain, they wanted to release me after the second day, but I opted for one extra day, which I was granted. When I was released they provided me pain pills to take home. I never used them. For all practical purposes the only discomfort was the catheter in me for 3 weeks after the surgery. After 3 days at home I was able to go to my office, carefully, and do about a 1/2 days work each day for the next few weeks. I followed instructions by performing my Kegel exercises 6 times a day to eventually gain control of my bladder urination. If the operation is successful, most men after the surgery are incontinent for any where from 4 months to a year. They will need to insert liners or absorbent guards/pads, which fit inside the shorts, until control comes back. The pads are available at most markets or drug stores.

The problem from the surgery is when the prostate is removed the inner sphincter is also removed, so pads are required until the muscles which make up the external sphincter are strengthend by continuously doing the Kegel exercises through contraction and relaxation of the pelvis floor muscles.

Initially, I had to change pads 5 to 6 times a day for the first 6 weeks and then my condition radically improved, so at the present time writing this chapter (my 5th month after the surgery), I am wearing only one pad a day and it appears I will be wearing no pads sometime real soon.

Six weeks after the surgery I was able to start playing golf and after 8 weeks I was back to my regular morning exercise running 2 miles every morning.

Three months after the surgery, I went for my blood test, which registered .05 PSA. Dr. Skinner said you are on your way. The last and most important concern was, will I be impotent the rest of my life. Dr. Skinner said, in your case, since you opted for the surgery at the very early stages of your cancer, with the nerves being spared, there is a good chance you will be normal for a 68 year old man, but it may take 10 months to a year. No doubt this is a “macho” concern for all men, but I feel quite confident because of the success of my procedure and catching it early I won’t have any problems.

In the future, I plan on a low fat diet rich in soy bean products, continue my exercise on a regular basis, avoid all stress related situations, go in every six months for a PSA blood test for the rest of my life, develop a better sense of humor by not taking life so seriously, enjoy my garden and pray daily to my God for the blessings he has bestowed upon me.

Summer, '04 is almost here, and it's been four and a half years since my Prostate surgery. Each year I have a scheduled check up by Dr. Don Skinner, my surgeon at the USC Norris Cancer Center and twice a year I see my attending physician Dr. Ram Nemani for PSA blood readings. So far my PSA readings have averaged 0.1 which is very comforting to me.

At the time, it was a major decision I had to make when I decided for the surgery over the other procedures. I feel in my mind I made the right decision. If there's cancer in an organ and I can remove it from my body without curtailing my normal functions, then I be that's the right way to go.

Before I decided on the surgery, I read Dr. Patrick C. Walsh's book "the Prostate - a Guide for Men and the Women who love them". By understanding the surgery procedure and the procedure Dr. Skinner described to me, I felt very comfortable with my decision and particularly confident in my surgeon being one of the best in the country.

The USC Norris Cancer Center was equipped with the proper up to date surgical devises to enable Dr. Skinner to preserve my bundle nerves. My cancer was in its very early stage, which made it easier to preserve the nerves.

My advise to everyone over fifty is to schedule a PSA blood test every six months in order to keep close watch on those PSA readings. I also advise everyone to establish a proper healthy diet, stay away from fatty foods, eat plenty of roughage (vegetables and salads) and grain foods, and drink at least six glasses of water each day. It is equally important to get into a routine exercise pattern. I go to the gym four times a week for about an hour of intensive workouts. God has been good to me, and for a 73 year old man, I am a very positive guy. I have always maintained a good sense of humor, and it was truly tested by my prostate problems. It is also vital that you go out of your way to avoid STRESS, as it will help you keep your body healthy. What better relaxing agent is there than laughing. It's therapy for our body. So keep happy and smell the roses!

My best to everyone for good health!

Chapter 22

THERE IS NO THEY

by William K. Weinstein

You've probably heard that when you get the word that it's cancer your life changes then and there, immediately, totally and possibly forever. Even if you've taken the time to think about it beforehand, until you've lived it, you can't really understand how much the words will mean and how totally consumed your life will become. Every thought you have, every feeling, every relationship is affected. You dream every night about dying from it and you realize very quickly that life going forward will never be the same. If you're like me you've probably never really questioned why the event would be so dramatic, the jolt so electric. It's unlikely that you'd ever analyzed what it is about our comfortable world that makes the discovery that you have cancer such an enormous event? Only when it actually happened to me and I suddenly felt like I was in a homemade canoe on a river rapidly approaching Niagara Falls, with no map, and just a small scrap of wood for a paddle, did I begin to understand.

It all began with a routine physical. My internist called with a generally good report card except that my PSA was somewhat high and should be followed. No reason to panic, just pay attention and get tested regularly. See a urologist, get his opinion, establish a relationship and stay tuned in. Then it all becomes gobbledygook for a year or so until I got the official pronouncement, an event that will be permanently embedded in my mind. I'll remember it in every detail for the rest of my life, just like where I was and how I reacted when Roosevelt died, JFK and Martin Luther King were shot, and when Chernobyl exploded.

I hadn't slept for two nights since undergoing my second biopsy and I had just arrived in my New York hotel room after a seemingly endless trip from home. I had willingly allowed the flight attendant to refill my wine glass as often as he wished to keep my mind from trying to predict or even contemplate the impending news. I showered and got dressed for dinner and only when no further diversions were possible did I finally dial my urologist in San Francisco to get the verdict. His receptionist put me on hold and there I stayed for twenty twilight zone minutes, my emotions alternating between despair, anxiety and a surging anger at the insensitive way I was being treated. If the news was good I wondered, wouldn't he have picked up right away? I was just getting ready to hang up and try to block the whole thing out of my mind until the next morning when my physician came on the line, vaguely apologized for keeping me waiting and informed me that it appeared I "had a little cancer". I was so strung out by then that I had to really strain to try to understand his words.

He was very sorry to have to give me the news. While this was certainly nothing to be taken lightly he thought it could be dealt with "adequately". I should make an appointment to see him as soon as I got back home. Did I have any immediate questions that I wanted to ask on the phone? Of course he needed to more carefully study my slides but there was no doubt that I had "frank cancer" on the right lobe of my prostate gland where nothing had shown up on the previous biopsy, three months earlier. On my left lobe where "atypia" (a condition in which some cells are observed to be abnormal and possibly suspicious) had been present on my first biopsy there was now evidence of PIN (prostatic intraepithelial neoplasia), a more advanced state of what is usually precancerous tissue change. I shouldn't panic, modern medicine had a good way to deal with prostate cancer and I was very fortunate indeed that he had discovered it when he did, so it could be properly treated. It's true that at age 56 I was quite young to have this disease but everything would probably turn out fine and the early diagnosis certainly stood me in good stead.

My Gleason grade (how close my cancer cells resembled normal cells), a very important component of both diagnosis and prognosis, was 2 plus 2 on a scale of 0 - 10, and my cancer had been staged at

T2B (a specific description of the character and extent of my tumor). He'd prefer to delay any further explanations until our appointment but I should try not to overreact (panic) until then. Most importantly, it would be wrong to assume that my cancer was growing very quickly just because the previous biopsy results had been completely normal on the right lobe, having shown no trace of disease, and, now, only a few months later, revealed cancer. "We must have just missed it last time". I should have a good time on my trip (right) and he would see me when I got back.

He was probably trying to make me feel better, but just thinking that he really might have missed it a few months earlier scared the hell out of me and incensed me even further. In a haze I left my hotel and since it had started raining and I had no chance of finding a cab on a wet New York street, I walked the fifteen or so blocks to my dinner appointment. About halfway there something totally unexpected happened. For the first time since this whole trauma had begun, I felt a sense of relief. Sure, I was very upset and quite frightened of what lay ahead, but, at some level, knowing the truth and no longer having to anticipate bad news, made me feel better. Something had snapped in me and I was sure I'd be able to deal with whatever I was about to face.

How wrong I was! What a fool I had been to react that way! Relief turned out to be an entirely inappropriate emotion. I had no idea how much confusion there is out there about prostate cancer or even a hint of the lack of knowledge, understanding or agreement that exists in modern medicine about how to deal with it. If I had understood the politics and economics that barricade the road to discovering what you have and what to do about it, I'd have gone umbilical right there on East 56th Street.

I was brought up to believe that when you get ill, you go to your physician who prescribes something or orders a particular treatment; then you get well. It had never occurred to me that I would suddenly be on my own with no real choice but to solve my crisis myself. I was being forced to become the captain of my own ship, facing decisions I felt hopelessly underqualified to make. And all this was happening in an unfamiliar and seemingly self-serving medical environment which I was finding to be generally user-unfriendly. The final choice was going to be mine to make only after battling my way through a maze of obstacles that were put up, perhaps inadvertently, by the very people who were supposed to be there to help. How could there be so little fact and such lousy data on a disease with so many victims, so broad an audience and such an endless daily supply of new participants?

This was my first revelation and the most important step every newly diagnosed man must take. You have to understand, accept and believe that even though your only qualification may be that you've driven past a medical school a few times on your way to work, in today's prostate cancer environment you have little choice but to take over total responsibility for your own life and proceed as best you can. You may find a physician who's friendly and comforting, but unless he's* one of the few truly well-informed and open-minded urologists out there, he can only be of limited assistance in making your decision and may even hinder it. Try as you may, you won't get beyond the point where you can make what a friend of mine calls "your most informed, best guess". You're not going to find universal truth because none yet exists. And, as you become really knowledgeable you may soon begin to suspect that you know considerably more about the disease than the urologist you're depending on. Not enough dialogue regularly takes place between physicians practicing various different approaches, so just sampling each one without bias gives you insight that most professionals won't have.

The sooner you accept this reality and learn to live and run with it, the better your chance of finding the answer that's right for you. When you get this part straight you'll understand that there is no

* Only about 2-3% of the urologists in the U.S. are women so I hope I'll be forgiven for using only the masculine pronoun throughout.

"they", only "you". You'll start to gain the power you're going to need to solve the mystery. When your friends ask: "what do they think?, what do they want you to do?, when are they going to decide?, what tests are they giving you?, and all the other typical they questions, you'll laugh to yourself, knowing that, in reality, they is really only you.

I found all this out the old fashioned way. When I got back home my search began immediately. Though the much anticipated appointment with my physician was very disappointing from the beginning, it was not unlike most of the sessions I would have with other urologists I later went to see. While each had its own set of particulars, they all sounded something like: 'we don't know anything for certain but our strong opinion is that surgery is the best answer for your disease. In medical school we were taught radical Prostatectomy** as the "gold standard" for prostate cancer. If it were me or my brother or father I'd cut the goddamn thing out and put it in a bottle where it belongs, where it can no longer hurt you. Yes there are other options but all of them are still highly experimental. We have more than 15 years of data on the results of radical Prostatectomy while they (the other modalities) have fewer than 10 years of outcomes. Surgery is the only procedure that really allows us to know where the cancer actually was (and wasn't) and how far it had actually progressed before it was removed. No other treatment choice provides that information, which can be very valuable later on, if your disease recurs.'

'If you do the proper thing, and choose surgery, I'd be happy to do it. I do the procedure as well as anyone else. Of course, I'm not Pat Walsh, the guy who gets all the media recognition. He invented "nerve-sparing" but we all do that now and he probably wouldn't take

---

** A radical Prostatectomy is the removal of the prostate, the seminal vesicles, and the lymph nodes around the prostate. The urine passage (urethra) is then reconnected between the bladder and that portion of the urethra beyond the prostate. A Prostatectomy takes from two to four hours to perform.

you anyway, because he only wants a sure thing, someone whose result is certain to improve his statistics. My primary mission is the removal of all your cancer. He wants to enhance his data with respect to potency (the ability to get a satisfactory erection) and continence (control of your urine). When I operate, I'll certainly try my best to make sure you aren't impotent or incontinent, but I'll take no shortcuts (no pun probably intended) to entirely eliminating your cancer and enabling you to reach your normal life expectancy, which at your age is what really counts. Walsh and his team often leave tissue in place to increase the probability of your not having one of those dreaded side effects but some of it could contain microscopic disease. I'm not even sure his published results are all that real because his patients are so anxious to please him that they fudge a little on their reports of sexual ability and urinary control. As for the operation itself, it typically takes me about 1 1/2 hours. Some other physicians take up to 4 hours, but I have no idea what they do in there for that long. The longer the surgery the more blood transfusions you're likely to require.'

When a urological surgeon gives you this speech he's really not whacking Walsh nor intentionally putting down the fabled "four hour man", Bill Catalona at Washington University in St. Louis, a urological surgeon known internationally for his pain-staking precision. He's just trying to win your business by assuring you of his competence. He's competing to gain your confidence so he can land you as a patient. As a general rule you'll find that the busier and more recognized the urologist, the less negative he is towards others in his field. But the collegial nature of the practice of urological medicine rarely survives the competition for a new surgical patient, especially one who seems willing or able to pay the financial price, usually \$20,000 - \$35,000.

Please understand that when I discuss the urological community I simply want to prepare you for the difficult environment you're likely to encounter and to warn you not to become complacent. I don't intend to demean it. These people are already beginning to feel like they're under siege and my comments are not likely to endear me or this article to them. More importantly, there's nothing to gain by alienating people who basically want to help and who claim to be trying to figure out how to best accomplish their goal. However, since the current reality doesn't always work in our best interest it has to be both well understood by the patient and constructively challenged, in the hope that we can cause rapid and dramatic improvement in time for all of us to benefit from it.

A retired urologist who is a dear friend of mine thinks that what's happened is really very clear. Urology's current plight is the culmination of a 15 year history of negative events which converged to make preservation of the highly remunerative radical Prostatectomy operation vital to the continuing economic stability of the profession and the individual physicians who practice it. 'First, we lost most of our surgery for kidney stones to lithotripsy', he explains, 'and then we watched as new medicines were introduced that largely replaced surgery for the treatment of BPH (benign prostate hyperplasia, a non-cancerous enlargement of the prostate gland). We've had a string of bad economic luck and while most of us are really pretty good people, not the awful cads some patients come to believe, radical Prostatectomy is a very attractive and profitable procedure for us. We enjoy performing the operation because it can be both complex and challenging and it really justifies our extensive and expensive medical school education's. Never underestimate how alluring all of this can be. Besides, if you'd been doing radical prostatectomies for 15 years, you'd be pretty upset if it turned out that you'd actually been harming the very people you were intending to help.'

It's hard to accurately describe the world such an attitude has created for the patient. Like me, you are likely to encounter what amounts to a conspiracy of silence, but not one crafted by diabolical or mean-spirited people. Rather, I discovered a network of physicians who honestly don't know the answers and have no reliable data on which to base their opinions. So, since its comfortable, profitable and convenient, they continue the well entrenched tradition of surgery. These physicians have to rely on flimsy and often outdated science, and unless a radical Prostatectomy is clearly contra-indicated they continue to perform it wherever applicable. They're observing the "golden rule" and most of the surgeons I've met genuinely believe that they're providing a real service. "If you don't have the data to reject my treatment method", they argue, "I'll do what I've been taught is best on as many people as I can help". Prostate cancer has hit the country in the form of an epidemic and many physicians simply say "I'm doing the best I can."

But are they? Regardless of their intent are they really accomplishing their stated goal? I found too many physicians who either weren't aware or just didn't want to discuss the substantial progress in alternative treatments that has occurred in the last few years. I feel passionately that not only should each patient be thoroughly acquainted with every viable treatment possibility, but I think he should be helped and encouraged by his physician(s) to conduct a really thorough search to find his own answer. Why should we be left on our own to try to create a path through an unfamiliar and very scary jungle?

A long-time friend of mine who works at a well known medical diagnostic company has just about lost his faith in the urology profession. His organization recently developed a product to help physicians better stage the extent of prostate disease in order to more precisely predict whether or not the cancer has remained within the prostate capsule, a very important factor in any decision about what treatment to choose. He's dumbfounded by the fact that only a tiny minority of the urological fraternity seems to have any interest in such a potentially pivotal piece of knowledge. He can't fathom why they don't want the added information the test may supply. His theory is that most of them don't want anything to disturb their comfortable worlds. Knowing too much might preclude them from proceeding in good conscience, so they continue to operate in a microcosm. They may not be aware of it but they are choosing confusion and doubt over knowledge. My friend has become so disillusioned that he's focused his product almost exclusively on the fast growing area of

Brachytherapy (radioactive interstitial seeding), where he's found an attitude of keen interest in anything that might help make a patient's diagnosis more accurate and predictive, the opposite response to the one he's generally received from the surgical community. His argument may even hint at certain malpractice issues on the part of some members of the urological community but my only interest is in the ultimate welfare of us patients.

In my quest for the "answer" I visited personally with thirty different physicians around the country and consulted by telephone and fax with fourteen more, including people in England, Sweden, Canada and Israel. And I interviewed at least as many patients as well as quite a few men who had chosen to take no conventional action of any kind to deal with their diagnosis, so-called "watchful waiters". Each professional I saw was reputed to be highly qualified and had the wallpaper to prove it. All the better ones, it turned out, were associated with major university hospitals1 and I still have plastic identification cards in virtually every color of the rainbow to remind me of my journey. The patients were men I heard about from friends and acquaintances, people who already had been forced to somehow deal with their prostate cancer, most of whom I found willing to open up and share their hearts with me.

My first "physician experience" was totally accidental but truly symbolic of what lay ahead. A close friend in Los Angeles knew I was flying down for a business meeting and urged me to arrive early. His wife has been fighting ovarian cancer for almost five years and he thought it would be helpful for me to talk to her two principal physicians. While they weren't prostate specialists they were both special people and highly regarded oncologists. He felt they could help me, so he set up a brief session with each of them. I had heard it was smart to bring someone with me to every meeting, not only for company but to make a record of everything that transpired and to help organize the information, so I asked my extraordinary assistant, Michiko, to join me. My strong advice to anyone who intends to have more than one or two medical examinations or interviews is to take along such a trusted friend, associate or spouse, someone who can take notes and help you remember the answers to your hundreds of nervous questions and collate the information to allow you to digest it better, when you're ready to review it and make your choice. If it's easier for you, tape the conversations and listen to the answers again at a more relaxed time. Spend as much time as you need organizing and re-thinking your most important concerns and questions. Today, when desperate men call me for advice and guidance, or when I'm not sure of what to do for myself, Michiko continues to play a key role as a result of her extensive experience and resulting expertise.

So, off we went to L.A. We met first with the senior member of the team, an internationally recognized gynecological oncologist and a warm and generous man. After reviewing my numbers and asking me a few questions, he confidently recommended that I have a radical Prostatectomy. He believed it to be the only definitive cure for cancer confined to the prostate, as mine appeared to be. Moreover, a man of my young (for this disease) age had to be directed toward that option which held the greatest promise of longevity. I got the "surgery as the gold standard" speech, the arguments that radiotherapy, etc. al. were not yet ready for primetime and a few similar points, all of which would soon become very familiar and which as a patient, you will get to know by heart. Then, just as he was concluding, his associate, my soon to be "second opinion", stuck her head in the room to remind him that his scheduled patients were backed up and waiting and he excused himself. Within five minutes, having examined the exact same data I'd just shown her senior partner, she confidently declared my choice to be "absolutely clear". "You must have radiation. Surgery is neither appropriate nor necessary for you." She told me who to see and where to go and advised me to be confident of a cure and get moving. It would be a shame if I chose surgery, it should be my "very last option". Then, she too had to get back to her patients; good-bye and good luck!

I was dazed. Here, within less than an hour, two recognized, distinguished and obviously interested physicians had earnestly expressed two diametrically opposing views about what was best for me, neither one knowing what the other had said. I felt like a character in a Kafka novel, but since this was virtually my first experience I had no idea how typical this encounter would be or how much more confused and disoriented my life would soon become. I had just started to look for an answer, but I had learned immediately that the journey was not going to be easy.

When we got back Michiko was able to get appointments with some of the people I needed to see in the East and in Chicago so we planned another trip. But I was already becoming a different person. I had done a few slightly smarter things since my diagnosis to better prepare myself and I was beginning to take control. I had completed three more medical visits in Los Angeles, including an appointment with Dr. Stuart (Skip) Holden, the medical director of CaPCURE (The Association for the Cure of Cancer of the Prostate). He was very helpful and, especially considering his surgery specialty, I found him quite open to other possibilities for treatment. He encouraged me to explore them all for myself. Not unexpectedly, he strongly favored Prostatectomy for all the standard reasons, though he was very realistic and forthcoming about its side effects. At my age, being divorced and interested in a new relationship, with no history of sexual problems, I had to face realistically the high possibility of impotence if I elected surgery. Incontinence wasn't terribly likely, but also had to be considered. I wouldn't have the rectal problems after surgery that I'd need to worry about if I chose any form of external beam radiation. True, the operation was a major one and it might take quite awhile for a full recovery but still, it was my best alternative. Brachytherapy was a possibility, but was not yet developed to the point where he could comfortably recommend it.

My meeting with Dr. Holden resulted from a call I had made to Mike Milken, someone I had known informally for many years because of his prominence in a field related to my business. He was very encouraging and supportive and immediately had his associate, CaPCURE Director Dr. Richard Atkins contact me to help map out a deliberate course of action. CaPCURE has made by far the greatest contribution of any organization to progress in prostate disease and we all owe it an enormous debt of gratitude and our continuing support. Not only has the organization raised $65 million to fund 450 prostate cancer related research projects worldwide (since 1993) but Mike, personally, has crusaded all over the country to raise awareness of the disease and the need to be regularly tested, particularly if you are a man over fifty or much earlier if there is any hereditary history of prostate cancer in your family. Say what you will about some of Milken's alleged behavior in the past, but there is no man alive whose untiring efforts and actions have meant as much to the current treatment and eventual cure of this disease. Mike is a real hero in this fight.

The other sane thing I had done to better prepare myself was to read Andy Grove's (Chairman of Intel) extraordinary article "Taking On Prostate Cancer" (Fortune, May 13, 1996). In retrospect, this should have been my first move and is absolutely required reading for anyone who is beginning the exploration process. Andy's article was a major factor in my coming to grips with the uncertainty I faced. He co-stars with Milken in this battle and has joined energetically in the effort to inform people about the disease and the many complications surrounding it. His discourse gave me perspective and really slowed down the urgency I had previously felt to make any decisions. And, at the same time, it legitimized my confusion.

One of the principal reasons that even the most accomplished medical people in the world begin every sentence about prostate cancer with the disclaimer that "no one knows for sure, but..." is because the data on this disease is both confused and incomplete. To group together a 50 year old in excellent physical condition in the same database with an 80 year old who's 50 pounds overweight and has been smoking cigarettes since he was 16 is patently ridiculous, but that's the state of the art. How can a scientific conclusion not account for factors like age, general health, prior history, heredity, lifestyle, socioeconomic status, vocation or other possibly relevant variables?

In the existing data, there has been almost no randomization, very few controls and the statistical endpoints for those studies that do exist are often not even remotely the same. So, the best you can say is that the results, sparse though they may be, are totally inconclusive. And, unfortunately, no matter how thorough your search, much of the data you uncover will end up being of little or no help. You just have to come to grips with this reality and accept it. Move on to your personal experiences with the brightest, most understanding and most knowledgeable people you can find. You really have no choice.

While Andy's article focused a lot on the science, it subtly raised the question of whether there actually can be a single conclusion that's right for everyone. What works for me, may not be right for you, emotionally or even physically. As I got to understand more about the whole area and the lack of solid data that exists, it became apparent that the more didactic, the more certain and more highly opinionated the medical practitioner, the less I could trust his opinion. Only those few who understood the lack of certainty surrounding the whole issue and took the time, interest and trouble to get to know what really makes a patient tick and matters most to him, turned out to be truly helpful. They were always the ones who were least defensive about the limits of their knowledge. They treated my journey with respect and encouraged and challenged me to continue the search and to let them know if I found anything that might expand what they clearly recognized to be the limits of their universe.

In addition to getting somewhat better informed, more focused and a little less scared, I had also given myself some time to get lucky. This is a very important element to remember because good fortune seems to happen more often if you provide it the opportunity. If you put your head down and blindly rush into something, you run the risk of precluding a lucky break. This time, mine came in the form of someone telling me that Dr. Dean Ornish of the Preventive Medicine Research Institute2 was just beginning a study to examine whether the principles he had established for treating heart disease many years earlier, might also work for cancer of the prostate. He hypothesized that the same general paradigm of nutrition, exercise, stress control and group support had a good chance to either control or actually cure the disease, so he was organizing a study using only those men who had already chosen watchful waiting, (about 20% of all American men who are diagnosed), as his patient population. Ethically this was the only place to get his participants since they had already independently decided against any conventional medical intervention. I knew Dean to be a caring and sensitive person whose refusal to accept mainstream thinking had changed and actually saved many heart victim's lives. So I called him to renew an acquaintance that had accidentally begun ten years earlier and he invited me to visit him in his office in nearby Sausalito. I was already leaning toward changing my eating habits since being impressed by my visit a week earlier with Dr. David Heber, the Director of UCLA's Center for Human Nutrition and I was very anxious for more information.

Dean could not have been more earnest or compassionate. He was beginning the trial because he really believed in its chances of success, but he had no hard evidence to present to me and wouldn't for at least a year. It might not work at all but if I wanted to try, he would let me join in a sort of special status, where I could participate freely and completely but my data wouldn't count in the overall results, since it would be unfair to other men who hadn't been able to get into the experimental group. I was invited to his retreat the following week. I could bring my former wife (one of my very best friends) as my supporting spouse and I could decide my future course of action without confounding his results, in case I continued down the road to a conventional therapy. He considered his approach to be a "serious and real intervention" and it was the one he would choose personally, were he in my situation. But, after a long interview with me, he understood my concern and confusion and would honor whatever decision I made. For sure he "wouldn't let those guys cut him up".

So, with really nothing to lose, I joined enthusiastically and got immediate benefits. I don't know if my cancer was in any way affected but my anxiety abated and my general health and happiness began the long trip back to where I so badly needed them to be. I experienced something entirely new and really enjoyed it. I had an instant support group, a new family of friends and we were living our crisis together. It taught me another very important lesson; don't stay alone with your problem for any longer than you can avoid. Don't hide it from your family or friends. To confront your crisis you need the best and biggest army you can gather so try to get over your hesitation and embarrassment and reach out for as much support you can muster. I dreaded having to tell my three incredible daughters that I had cancer and I procrastinated as long as I could, but once it was done I had the strongest allies anyone could hope for. Also, I suggest you join a support group like Peter Korda describes in his book, Man To Man, another piece of mandatory reading. Mine meant an incredible amount to me, giving me love and understanding and a chance to share my fears and issues with people who were in the same condition as the one in which I suddenly found myself.

I realize that the advice to go public with your problems may ignore some very complicated work-related issues as well as some very real potential medical insurance concerns that may loom for you. However, I really believe you should make every possible effort to overcome these issues to satisfy your other legitimate needs. Get mad if you have to, but don't let the bastards beat you down. Defiance is a much better posture for men with this disease than denial or passive acceptance. Make the problem theirs: the employers, insurers, or any other organization threatening to make your life even harder, many of whose senior decision makers are unfortunately very likely to be diagnosed with this same disease within the next few years. The many horror stories I've heard from other patients have convinced me that to turn the other cheek and be polite is a crummy idea with bad ramifications for all of us. You may have to fight hard for your rights but every blow will be a big help to all of us.

After Dr. Ornish explained how the high animal fat and animal protein present in "normal American diets" helped cancer proliferate and grow and showed me lots of evidence in animals which demonstrated that eliminating most fat from the diet seemed to starve the disease and drive it toward the baseline of dormancy, I reluctantly gave up my previous eating habits and became a vegan vegetarian. I've rarely cheated since then and I'll probably try to maintain this kind of nutritional program for the rest of my life. I believe strongly that sharply curtailing your fat intake is a smart adjunct to any other form of therapy you ultimately choose and that most afflicted men will benefit a lot from giving it a try. It can also be a very good discipline to practice for prevention of the disease, if you begin early enough.

For me the diet and the exercise parts of the overall Ornish intervention were much easier than the stress control programs, which I just couldn't get used to. No yogi in the world need fear any competition from me. But I did give it a real try and I have kept it up fairly regularly since then. I learned some yoga poses and although I don't practice daily I try to meditate for at least 5-10 minutes, 3-4 times a week. I think that merely attempting to control your stress is a large part of the battle and no matter how bumbling you might be, trying is succeeding. In any event, however I got there I had spent over a month working with my fear and I was now in much better physical and emotional shape to go forward. I was more secure, I felt better and I was more ready in general for what I needed to do on my next trip.

When I got to New York my first appointment was with a physician at a famous Manhattan hospital complex, whom I later came to regard as a true buffoon. He gave me a very rough and impersonal general examination and then, looking directly at the written summary of my pathological results which I'd brought along with me, and using a very painful finger, proceeded to try to make me his patient by scaring the hell out of me. He was the first (and only) physician to describe my tumor as a large mass and one that could be easily moved around, neither of which are favorable. In a very superior sounding voice he told me "We do it all here; radical prostatectomies, external beam radiation, seeds, you name it. We're expert at all of them so all you have to do is decide which one you want and my nurse will schedule you!" His entire demeanor was designed to suggest that only he could save my life.

When I finally got out of his office I had to physically restrain myself from running, full speed, to my next appointment so I could find out what the hell was going on. Had my cancer suddenly changed character? Was it growing out of control? I was on my way to Memorial Sloan-Kettering, the Cancer Temple, to see one of the few people who specialize in prostate oncology in the entire country. There are only a handful I would unconditionally recommend and you will probably end up having to rely upon the opinions of a variety of other specialists for this function, if you want to reach beyond the typical urologist for consultation. Until more oncologists are trained to understand the specific characteristics and problems of prostate disease, you will have to make the best of an imperfect situation and be creative. Get the best opinions you can from wherever you can find them and try to stay away from those people who start out with a strong singular bias. Seek professionals who have a true overview who can help you objectify the choices and put the whole question into reasoned perspective.

Dr. Howard Scher, thankfully was my next appointment. He focuses his practice mainly on advanced prostate disease but he has an especially sharp mind and a special ability to help move you toward a decision. He seems to understand the confusion and disillusion that's out there for us. He and his "medical fellow", a younger disciple to whom he was teaching the trade, both examined me digitally (finger), believe it or not at my request. I had been so frightened by my previous visit I just had to know if my cancer had suddenly gone crazy. It was only after neither of them could find much of note in my tumor that I was finally able to relax a little from the mean scare the other guy had just thrown into me an hour earlier.

After some general conversation, Scher stated his preference for surgery in my case because of the localized nature and early diagnosis of my disease, the small size of my tumor, and because of my age.

But, like the other diagnosticians I saw or spoke with on my journey who had no specific ax to grind and nothing personal to gain, he felt that the most important thing was that I "do something". To him, it mattered a whole lot less exactly which therapy I chose, than that I at least opted for one of the conventional treatments, rather than "watchful waiting and doing nothing".

There is enormous controversy over this point and you should really understand it. After I finally finished my due diligence process a couple of months later, I spent a difficult and uncomfortable two weeks pondering this very question, before making my final decision. There are very, very few practicing urologists in the United States who would regularly recommend watchful waiting to a man under 70 years old. But this is true exclusively in America. By contrast, there are not many physicians in other countries around the world who routinely recommend surgery. Watchful waiting is by far their most frequent prescription, but were they to suggest any actual procedure at all it would likely be some form of radiation, a less intrusive process with a far easier and speedier recovery. American medicine has made enormous strides in many key areas, but there are a number of highly respected scientific centers in other countries whose medical views should also be considered.

Most of the physicians I saw or spoke to cited my age as the key factor in their recommendation for surgery. I was regularly told that only if I were 70 or older would the option of doing nothing be a viable one and even then it might not be right. Certainly, at that age, surgery should only be employed under special circumstances. However, when you look at the actual practice of urologists in the United States, a much higher percentage of older men than you would expect are regularly being subjected to the knife, possibly unnecessarily sentenced to a far less enjoyable existence than necessary, for the rest of their time on this planet.

Surgeons "cut" and many seem to sincerely believe th□□at's why they were born. They havto exude confidence to successfully solicit patients so they'd better believe in what they do. A urologist is a surgeon by training, so when you're referred to one you are asking a question of a biased respondent, usually one who is totally committed to his training, and often, as I've indicated, shockingly unaware of the rest of the medical world and it's differing points of view. Certainly, these people have been extensively educated, but think about what they've been taught. They got through medical school, though mainly not at the heads of their class, primarily by learning to memorize and to do things by rote. Originality, creativity and special inventiveness were discouraged and possibly even punished. Upon graduation, when their commitment to the knife as the final adjudicator was complete, they were sent out into the world to pronounce their pre-ordained judgments upon those of us unlucky enough to need them.

As I witnessed this firsthand, I quickly became guilty of the same heresy hinted in Dr. Grove's article. And the boys heard well his implied threat to their security and have circled their wagons in response. Quite a few of the physicians I saw went out of their way to be very solicitous about his intent, but they couldn't believe how "unsound" his conclusion was, given his own discovery of the lack of data that exists. "Poor Andy", they confided, "hadn't listened to his own advice". One highly publicized surgeon at a major clinic in the Midwest went so far as to exclaim, unsolicited, that "if Andy Grove ran Intel the way he's running his medical life, the company would be bankrupt by now". This is the same physician who diagnosed me over the telephone, without ever having seen me or my pathology slides and after having talked with me for less than fifteen minutes. He told me unequivocally that I needed an operation and I'd best make an appointment with him as soon as possible so he could get it done.

Andy, for his part, told me that he's received more than 1,500 communications since writing his treatise and that "no one has been able to give me information that would change my mind". In his view, the "dice were loaded". The data comparing surgery with other modalities took all the surgical rejects, those who were beyond the point where surgery was an option and lumped them into the opposing (non-surgical) numbers. These men were, by definition, much sicker, so placing them into the opposing sample naturally made surgery look much better than it actually is. But, if you adjust this standard error out to more fairly compare apples to apples, the radiation group does at least as well and arguably even better than those men who had surgery, at equivalent time periods. At best it's a difficult and speculative exercise but the superiority cited by surgeons for their treatment is indefensible and it would be nice if more of them conveyed that message clearly and honestly to their patients. Don't be so naive as to expect it, but insist that your physician show you the latest data, not just the convenient comparisons from four years ago, before much of the current information came to light. And while you're at it, demand information about his own individual surgical results so you can compare it to others when you try to determine who to use. Find out what results he's had, particularly in the areas of incontinence, impotence and recurrence. Remember these people are being introduced to the concept of accountability for the first time. Their patients want proof and are suddenly questioning every aspect of their advice, as well they should.

The person I saw next is perhaps one of the most intriguing men I've ever met. His name is Zvi Fuks and he ran the Department of Radiation Oncology at Memorial Sloan-Kettering, in the same complex as Howie Scher, whose office I'd just left. His presence is magical and he immediately makes you comfortable. His point of view is very definite, but, because he knows how to listen, not as didactic as many of the other professionals I met. He exudes intelligence and power and is certainly one of the best informed people anywhere about the challenges and possibilities that currently exist in prostate cancer. His chosen field, three dimensional conformal external beam radiation therapy (3D XRT) is certainly one to consider and is being used in many advanced centers around the world. Fuks is one of the undisputed leaders in the field of radiation therapy.

After reviewing my data and pathology slides and giving me my fourth digital rectal exam in as many hours, Zvi invited me to sit down and "get serious". The pathologist my urologist had chosen to do my Gleason scoring was an amateur and my grading was too low. It was probably a 6, (3+3) worse than the (2+2) 4 I had been told, but not necessarily something to get frightened about. Gleason's, it seems, are widely interpretable and can vary substantially, especially amongst physicians who don't do them everyday. However, every man who is diagnosed with prostate cancer is given his Gleason grading and it strongly influences the decision of what or what not to do. One of the scariest parts of the whole puzzle is witnessing the inability of the profession to standardize something so widely quoted and influential in your final choice. I strongly urge you to get at least two opinions as to what your Gleason grade is and possibly more. Don't assume that every pathologist really understands the process. Many don't. A second opinion from another professional is easily obtained from the same slide, without another biopsy.

A grade of Gleason 6, Zvi explained, is not a Gleason 7, the point at which both the diagnosis and the prognosis often change negatively, sometimes significantly. He thought my tumor type was a T1C, a slightly different classification than that given by my original urologist. It described a mass which is small and really not palpable. With a Gleason 6 and a PSA of less than 10, mine was a "good tumor". He put my chance to be cured at a very happy 90% and reduced the possible ways for me to go to three: 3D conformal radiation, seed implants, and, of course, surgery. In his view, the seeding exposure might be a bit more toxic than I needed, and some percentage of it was too "blind" for him but if I elected it anyway I should expect exactly the same potential cure rates as I would with surgery or with 3D XRT. Then, the preliminaries having been dispensed with, he launched into a comprehensive description of his specialty and why I might want to consider it for my disease.

3D XRT electronically re-constructs the inside of your body so that the x-ray therapy team can see with extraordinary precision exactly where the x-ray beam is going, in a number of simultaneous fields. In this way the prostate can be programmed for radiation that is much stronger than can be delivered by the standard external beam method, without increasing the risk of damage to surrounding organs and tissue, principally the immediately adjacent rectum and bladder. The dosage can be raised quite high, (for me it would be 81 gy), so as to maximize the possibility for successful ablation of the cancer. I would need a total of 45 sessions, approximately 1/2 hour a day, 5 times a week for 9 weeks. The procedure would be performed by a team which he would lead. My chances of impotency after 3D XRT he put at 30%, the same odds he believed I'd have in the hands of "the best surgical operators, like Pat Walsh". He predicted my likelihood of long-term incontinence to be 0% after 3D XRT versus about 5-10% after surgery, a number which I now believe to be more accurately 5-25%, if your definition of continence is normal and complete urinary control. Rectal complications, of which there was almost no likelihood after surgery, did sometimes accompany his treatment, but rarely did they require anything more than a simple remedy, like Preparation H.

Overall, Zvi favors his treatment methodology because he believes it provides the greatest degree of control. He thinks he can eliminate the cancer equally well without damaging anything around it, with much less wear and tear on the patient than surgery. He compared this "recovery factor" in the average patient as follows: a man usually becomes slightly less physically active for 9-12 weeks while undergoing 3D XRT and may possibly remain a bit tired for a short period when it's over. After surgery most men have significantly reduced energy for a couple of months and don't feel really normal for a year or more. With seeds you're "done in one day but you could be sick for months", dealing with the inevitable discomfort of urinary frequency and urgency.

Zvi is very passionate in his beliefs about the superiority of 3D XRT. He's demonstrated his conviction by treating five of his closest friends with this procedure, something he confided he never would have done were he not totally convinced both of its efficacy and comparative advantage over other choices. All five, he told me, were successes, at least so far, and he was optimistic about their chances for not suffering recurrences.

While he taught me a lot and generally prepared me to be a much smarter patient, one of the most important contributions he made to my knowledge base was his refutation of the "myth" promulgated by a majority of the urologists I interviewed. One of the strongest reasons they gave for recommending surgery over radiation is that once the prostate is radiated there is so much scar tissue created that if surgery does become necessary at a later date, it is rendered either difficult or impossible because the surgeon can't precisely distinguish the cancer from other tissue. When I tried this thesis out on Zvi, he pulled himself up to his considerable height, got a very angry look on his reddening face and screamed "that's Bullshit!" a number of times. He then proceeded to review with me the results he was aware of for sixteen patients who had been operated on successfully in the past twelve months, three to five years after receiving 3D conformal radiation. He cited personal experience with cases in which radiation may actually have made prostate surgery easier to perform, rather than "virtually impossible". He definitely takes a very dim view of the misinformation many patients regularly receive. Overall, he was an enormous help and I left feeling much more ready to understand and evaluate what was to come and knowing that there was at least one seriously viable alternative to surgery. I have subsequently spent some time on the whole issue of salvage therapies and I now believe that a Prostatectomy under these circumstances would not be a first choice anyway. There are a number of alternatives already available and more to come in the near future, a fact which further reduces the potential negative of radiation as a primary choice.

The next day I headed for Baltimore to see the most famous prostate physician of them all. This is the man who recently stated on a national news program that the problem with prostate surgeons is that many of them don't really know what they're doing and consequently are just "practicing on their patients". There I was, with "The Man", Dr. Patrick Walsh, the inventor of nerve sparing surgery, known all over the world for his competence and creativity. Though I had been told to expect an arrogance that for him alone should be endured, I actually encountered a pleasant and congenial person who seemed quite anxious to explain the prostate cancer world to me, and did so in a measured and surprisingly patient way. Dr. Walsh, you see, owns Johns Hopkins; it's his and he knows it. He's the undisputed king of radical prostatectomies, a title he wears on his forehead, not in conceit, but rather in total self-confidence. When he speaks you find yourself grateful for every word and since you know beforehand how selective he is in choosing patients you're trying harder to impress him and make him like you than vice versa.

He quickly informed me that he insists on interviewing each patient personally, that he performs every surgery himself and that he gives each patient his home phone number and wants them to feel free to contact him at any time. He also offered to provide some patient references, with their prior permission. We went through my various scores and staging and he reviewed my biopsy slides and the accompanying interpretation. He, too, immediately dismissed my Gleason scoring. It was too low—probably a 5 or 6, not a 4 as my pathologist had said. He examined me digitally, typed me and after describing the extent of my tumor pronounced me a "perfect candidate", to my total delight. I had made the cut (pun intended) and for a short moment I was truly happy for the first time since being diagnosed. Dr. Patrick Walsh was willing to operate on me.

He believed that the only other serious option for me to consider was 3D XRT since he considers interstitial seeding (or Brachytherapy) to be "still experimental" and in general, he too, was very encouraging about my chances for a cure. Even if the cancer has penetrated the wall of the prostate you can still cure it, he explained. People with positive lymph nodes may not be really curable, but those whose cancer has spread into the seminal vesicles are. He reiterated the generally accepted thinking about what most men should opt to do: If you're 40 to 60, have surgery; 60 to 70, it's not clear, except perhaps in specific individual cases; over 70, choose radiation. A bit simplistic perhaps, but informative nonetheless.

Then he encouraged me to ask questions and his answers were very concise: "Don't even think about my operating on you if you use hormones first. Surgery is certainly the best treatment if the tumor is confined to the prostate. For men in their 50's, the overall potential for potency after my surgery is 75%, your chances are 60-75%, depending on whether or not I have to take out a nerve bundle, which I won't know until I operate. Incontinence isn't a real concern after I operate, so don't worry about it." He repeated his view that radiation is preferable only for men over 70. Watchful waiting will result in the lesion growing outside the prostate and eventually metastasizing. Cryosurgery (freezing the cancer to death) is "outrageous, done right the impotency rate is 100%".

Dr. Walsh allowed that sex would definitely be different after surgery. But he was the first person to dispel one of my greatest fears, one that derived from my ignorance of the meaning of impotency. He carefully explained that even if I were to be unlucky and be rendered impotent after my operation, it would have no physical influence on my sex drive. Impotency only describes one's ability to get an erection sufficient for intercourse. He assured me that sexual sensation would be present and that I would probably be able to have an orgasm even without the ability to get a normal erection, since they derive from your brain, not your penis. I might have to use one or more of the new products on the market (Viagra, MUSE, Caverject) to achieve an erection if that was important to me or my partner, but, in any event, I should be able to reach a sexual climax. The actual event would not be exactly the same since there would be no ejaculate and many men had described the sensation of orgasm as flowing inward, not outward as before. Nonetheless they were having a sexual release and were generally satisfied.

Then he got somewhat carried away and told me that I really shouldn't worry about it anyway because a number of people recently had reported to him that "sex was actually better now, after surgery." Better, I asked, to make sure my ears were working, wondering what the hell he was talking about. He sparkled, and said something to the effect that when it's less frequent and takes a lot longer, it can be more of an event. Spontaneity isn't everything. Sometimes, if it requires better planning, and more assistance, it can be more meaningful, especially it seemed, for the women in his sample.

I later thought about this part of the conversation and decided that having God-like hands is enough, you don't have to be totally logical or sensible in every aspect of your thinking to be a truly great surgeon. And think about the kind of commitment to one's point of view it takes to fervently promote your position with a curious argument like the "sex is better now" concept. Dr. Walsh is completely certain about what he does everyday and totally believes in himself and that's undoubtedly an important part of what makes him so special. But, in spite of his recently televised comments about his peers, and his apparent concern for the reality that most patients encounter, the fatal flaw is that his published comments and recommendations seem to somehow assume that his genius is generally available to all of us. He doesn't seem to fully understand that the surgical world most men encounter is nothing like his. Somehow, he can't grasp the unpleasant reality that confronts many of the patients of most of the 8,500 other urologists "practicing" in the United States. And, it's not even totally clear that Walsh's own excellent results are repeatable in any but a carefully chosen and generally unrepresentative sample of the current patients in today's prostate cancer universe.

There are a few other extraordinary surgeons around the country, but, in my view, only a few. If I chose to be operated on, there are fewer than 25 urologists I would seriously consider. If I couldn't gain access to one of them or someone they recommended whom I had thoroughly investigated, I simply wouldn't choose surgery and, unless things change, neither should you. It's not that lots of other urologists aren't competent. They just don't have anywhere near the same level of knowledge, commitment or experience. Their facilities aren't as good and they don't have available to them the same support from other competent specialists. Often they have no university affiliation in which to maintain constant up-to-the-minute awareness and other professionals to talk and share experiences with. And, they don't spend the same significant portion of their waking lives teaching and learning, traveling all over the continent in pursuit of each new potential treatment or possible cure that arises.

Almost all of the physicians in my small group are not only top-flight surgeons but are also people who have a deep knowledge and appreciation of the vagaries of prostate cancer and who are willing to openly discuss and consider other alternatives with you. Some, like Fuks and Walsh, have singular points of view, but they are derived with genuine integrity. Most of them are actively engaged in research on possibilities beyond surgery or whatever their chosen specialty. Unfortunately, they are amongst the very few in whose hands we should feel comfort and confidence.

This whole issue has become even more complex and disturbing for many patients because of the trend towards managed care. Not only have their choices been substantially reduced, but I am suspicious of any process that somehow automatically confers acceptability on whatever is done internally, within the microcosm of the organization. I've heard from a number of men who are participants in programs like Kaiser's, or other similar HMO's, that they feel pushed down a pre-determined path and actively discouraged from seeking alternatives. If they choose to follow a convenient transition from internist to urologist and into surgery they're pretty well covered, though neither physician may be particularly skilled or experienced. If, however, they want to explore different arenas, they feel thwarted, especially, it seems, if they choose no conventional therapy at all. The very system which should profit from less expensive alternative choices seems challenged by it. In any case, as with the whole medical apparatus in our country, the managed care providers either must quickly get far more skilled in handling prostate disease or they will experience some very serious strains. Men are finally speaking out and demanding a much higher level of care and the system is beginning to hear the message.

As I've tried to convey, my conclusion that "there is no they" came very reluctantly and only after considerable personal experience. At one point, I thought about charging admission to anyone who wanted to give me a digital rectal exam, many of which I believe were either unnecessary or performed by people who had very little idea of what they were looking for. Unsympathetic, uneducated fingers hurt and you don't need to submit to just anyone who pretends to a title. Also, the prostate gland does not readily reveal itself in its entirety, often leaving much of its surface concealed. If many of the prostate specialists I saw couldn't do it right, pity the poor internist or other gatekeeper who may be causing pain and embarrassment with very little diagnostic justification.

I believe that this whole process needs to be re-thought. It may be keeping more men away from being examined than the value of the diagnoses it produces. Very few prostate cancers are discovered this way today and when they are, it's often too late anyway. Some physicians argue that although they agree that the finger examination shouldn't be the first line of defense against cancer of the prostate, it can frequently discover rectal or colon cancer and therefore should be encouraged, an argument I certainly respect. But, if a very important key to successful treatment is early diagnosis, then somehow making the process much less frightening and finding a compromise which minimizes our anxiety is vital to getting us to submit ourselves for examination on a regular basis. At the very least a whole new approach must be considered. For some reason the medical profession just hasn't gotten the message.

The PSA (prostate specific antigen) blood test, imperfect as it may be, is by far our best hope at the moment. Since it is the only real marker available, its intelligent and proper usage has to be actively encouraged and promoted by the profession to every man over a given age and certainly to anyone with a family history. It will help you personally to remember that your results may vary substantially from one test to the next so try to help yourself achieve the lowest number possible: Don't let your physician examine you digitally before a PSA, the blood must be drawn before pulling your pants down for the finger examination; don't have sex of any kind for 72 hours prior to your PSA appointment; and, although this is more controversial, I wouldn't ride a bike or do anything particularly physical that might somehow stimulate the prostate for a few days before getting tested.

After a discovery of prostate cancer is made by the PSA, a digital exam is certainly appropriate, but in my view, rarely vice versa. Moreover, there are a number of additional tests which can add measurably to the diagnostic process available today as well as some other diagnostic systems currently in clinical trials, any of which potentially could be more accurate than the PSA. So getting men to be willing to be regularly tested, and to actually do so voluntarily will become even more critical to controlling this epidemic when we find a more reliable marker. I've discussed my point of view with a number of prominent pros and while they don't necessarily dispute my basic premise, they insist that once the diagnosis is established a finger exam helps them plan the details of the procedure they're about to perform. We can certainly live with that.

Anyway, after being anointed by Walsh, I flew from Baltimore to Chicago for two more consults and a short visit with my closest friend. Even though both physicians I saw there tried hard to be helpful, it was basically more of the same. Yes, the surgery is very difficult to endure and the published side effect numbers are too optimistic, but it couldn't possibly be as bad as you're hearing. It's the best thing we have right now. Since you're too young to do nothing, and we can't find anything better, you have no choice. Surgery is best employed as your first option because if you have to elect it as a salvage procedure you're almost certain to be impotent and highly likely to be incontinent, etc., etc., etc.

So, although they didn't have much to add to my stewing pot, like everywhere else I went I got some new information that could potentially be very helpful. One of the physicians I saw specialized in the study and treatment of impotence. While urging me to have the surgery he gave me a strong suggestion that he thought would increase the chances of maintaining my potency after the operation. Right after the catheter's removed, in approximately 4-6 weeks, it's smart to encourage erections on a regular basis. Viagra wasn't yet approved and its impact might be too systemic but I could use a device known as MUSE to achieve the desired localized result. Just place it inside the urethra and release a small pellet of a safe, naturally occurring substance called alprostadil or if I preferred, I could get the same result using Caverject, an injection of alprostadil directly into the penis. Pick whichever one I liked best but use it often, even though I may not be having actual sexual intercourse for awhile, because having blood flowing into my penis and getting muscle memory re-established would increase my chances of regaining potency. This whole concept made a lot of sense to me and I've since heard it from enough people I respect to recommend it to the attention of anyone who elects surgery, or, possibly after any other alternative therapy that compromises or threatens one's ability to get an erection.

The other lesson I received on this visit was an open acknowledgment that the term "incontinence" is used very differently by urologists in various centers and practices around the country. To some physicians it means what I think it should; not having total control over your urine. But many others get cute and define it as having to change a sanitary pad in your undershorts less than three times per day. Be absolutely certain that you understand exactly what your physician means when he discusses the likelihood of incontinence with you. Be sure you're both talking about the same thing. Remember, it's you who will have to deal with this problem, physically and psychologically, so you'd better fully understand it. You also should discuss "stress incontinence", to be able to accurately anticipate the likelihood of leaking when doing whatever your favorite physical activity is, after surgery. If you wet yourself each time you take a backswing before hitting a golf ball, or return a serve or hit a triple, or you're going to have to carry dry shorts along on your three mile jog, you should at least be aware of these possibilities and be able to consider them carefully before you decide what to do.

After these two sessions, I retreated to the comfort of my friend's home to regroup and as we talked I began to realize how unsatisfied I was becoming with a lot of the advice I was getting. The physicians I had seen seemed, for the most part, to be decent guys, just doing what they perceived to be their jobs, pushing me toward what they'd been taught was right and would be paid handsomely to perform. But for me it just wasn't clicking. I couldn't get my heart or my stomach to swallow the stuff that was pummeling my brain. In the process of trying to describe my frustration and confusion to my friend of 20 years, I realized that I was going to have to go even further. Although I had already gained a great deal of information I'd need to do more research, see more people and reach out in every direction I could think of. We agreed that I would go crazy if I didn't decide on something quite soon and I promised him that I would do just that. Although I really didn't know what that would be, we both sensed that I was becoming fairly certain of what it wasn't.

When I got back home, we again broadened the search for other treatment possibilities and once again, largely through Mich's persistence, had good fortune. She succeeded in arranging appointments with two unusually thoughtful and highly sought after physicians in our own backyard, at UCSF in San Francisco. Dr. Peter Carroll is the Professor and Chair of the Department of Urology and therefore has responsibility for the entire universe of approaches to the prostate cancer problem being tried at the university. Each distinct modality reports to him, requiring that he know a great deal about every area and that he remain open to progress, wherever it may occur. All the grant applications and other money raising efforts in each sub-specialty must be approved and encouraged by him so his breadth of knowledge and willingness to consider a range of therapies is an absolute prerequisite. He seems the right person for the job because he's been able to put the typical medical school mentality behind him and open his mind to today's fast-changing environment. He understands well that an approach of any kind which has a serious chance of changing the course of this disease is one worth pursuing.

Carroll questions everything, while remaining open to anything. He seems comfortable in each alternative arena and is not married to any one approach, though he does practice urological surgery. Perhaps it is this non-defensive willingness to explore and consider any plausible alternative that has enabled him to attract so many outstanding people and why his UCSF department is today recognized as one of the finest. It may also be why I felt so immediately comfortable with him. Quality of life is a primary consideration to him, not a footnote, and though he believed my perception of the negative consequences of prostate surgery to be overblown, he totally acknowledged and supported my concerns. After going over my personal data with me he fielded my many questions and addressed them with sensitive candor.

As a general proposition for a person with a small and encapsulated tumor, he wasn't sure hormone treatment (the chemical equivalent of castration) prior to another procedure really would help, but it probably wouldn't hurt. There may be a synergistic impact, particularly in large volume disease, though there is no established benefit in small volume disease, like mine. If I were to elect to use it I should not opt for a long term antigen deprivation course and I should seriously question my motivation in considering it altogether. Was I afraid that seeds might not work in the long term and if so why was I contemplating going that route? Similarly, did I doubt that 3D XRT would provide a lasting cure and wasn't a hormonal blockade simply a way to hedge my bet? The issue for me to consider should be whether either of these, or any other methodology would be equivalent to surgery, without the high risk of problems afterward. While hormones will definitely reduce the volume of the prostate and your PSA score, you must decide whether you need that benefit enough to risk the side effects, which may differ considerably from patient to patient. Or, as another physician said to me "I know of no insurance policy for which you don't have to pay a premium. Any additional treatment you choose to combine with another will have the potential of increased cost in the form of a greater possibility of producing a more negative side-effect profile". Peter concluded "I remain neutral. If you aren't afraid of the possible problems, it can't hurt, but I'm not convinced it helps either".

He pointed out that there are lots of new concepts coming, both therapeutic and diagnostic. "There's recently been some real progress in vaccines, especially of the dendritic variety, both here at UCSF and with Dr. Gerald Murphy's group in Seattle, which might strongly influence a man's decision in the next few years. 'If we had a salvage therapy that had a high probability of working it would make your initial choice much easier and less filled with anxiety.' Having a fall-back position more desirable than salvage radical Prostatectomy would make an "informed gamble" based on quality of life factors a less scary proposition and an easier choice because if it ultimately failed you could always try another therapy with a high probability of subsequent success.

We discussed a number of other diagnostic tests, including the experimental MR Spectroscopy being developed at UCSF to better assess the activity of one's tumor which I had just undergone and concluded that while any of them might be helpful, none were yet far enough developed to be so singularly significant in my process as to really dictate my decision. Any additional information they might generate could always help, but Peter felt that I already knew enough of the basics and I should now focus on the more exacting particulars of the choices I was down to. He seemed to intuitively sense that surgery wasn't going to make me happy and he believed that if I chose it, my heart wouldn't be in it. So he strongly advised me to eliminate surgery as a possibility and concentrate on which form of radiotherapy would be best for me. "Basically you have to make a decision and stick to it. You have to be comfortable with it before, during and after it's done!" He was pleased to learn that I was about to see his associate, Mack Roach, head of Urological Radiotherapy at the university to get his point of view, and he also confirmed that heading north to Seattle to explore the Brachytherapy universe was a good idea and that I should get going. I was encouraged by his sense that I was close to the point where I would feel it all come together and that the choice would soon become clear to me.

Dr. Roach is a very considered, hard-working and deliberate person, and one of the few I found who has maintained perspective and a sense of humor while remaining passionate about what he does and the patients he treats. He was happy to help analyze every issue I raised, in whatever level of detail I required, to help make my thinking process clearer. He was especially helpful in explaining the puzzle I was trying to solve; comparing results between the various major treatments. He focused me squarely on the fact that the data being presented at meetings he had recently attended showed no significant difference between any of them. 3D XRT, proton radiotherapy (a different form of radiation), Brachytherapy, and surgery all seem to be producing the same probability of near term treatment efficacy, measuring from 1 to 8 years. "You run into difficulty going further out because of the lack of data." One of the basic problems he suggested I might be having in making direct comparisons was probably being created by each specialist's lack of real insight into any treatment area other than his own. Everyone seemed to be keeping his head down, focusing entirely on his own special interest and not worrying about the others. The brachy guys really didn't understand the trials and tribulations of surgery, the surgeons didn't know much about 3D XRT, etc. There was almost no cross-fertilization so most specialists couldn't really help a patient's thinking about any other modality.

Mack, however, had no trouble understanding my lack of enthusiasm for surgery and reinforced it by citing the results of a number of studies showing an extremely high percentage of cancer recurrence after surgical removal of the prostate gland. His skepticism was undoubtedly influenced by the large number of patients in his practice who required radiation shortly after a "successful" Prostatectomy, or later, when the cancer reappeared. He believes passionately in 3D XRT, but isn't at all closed to other alternatives and has recently begun to use radioactive seeds in his practice. Also, he's doing some experimenting with combinations of primary therapies. I'm not sure whether it was his sense of fairness or his basic conservatism that came through when I asked him what he would do in my position. He thought about it for a while and said "I'd do a short hormonal gig, follow it with some 3D XRT and then I'd get seeded". In other words follow three non-surgical routes, all in moderate dosages. Rather than try to pick one solution, hedge your bet. I didn't follow all his advice in the end but his careful explanations and genuine interest helped me a lot and prepared me well for my next excursion.

I was on the plane again, this time with appointments to see both Dr. Timothy Mate, Andy Grove's coveted physician, and Dr. John Blasko, both of whom practice up in Seattle. I'd spoken to Grove about Mate and I'd also heard terrific things about Blasko, including his getting much of the credit for bringing the treatment technique known as interstitial seeding or Brachytherapy back to life and up to it's present level of efficacy. Both men are pioneers and though they are radiation oncologists, not urologists, they possess tremendous knowledge about prostate cancer and most of the current possibilities for treating it.

I never got to know Mate as well as I would have liked because he didn't think I was a good candidate for his particular approach, called HDR (High Dose Radiation) in which radioactive "smart bombs" are inserted into the prostate for short intervals, usually over a two-three day period. They do not remain in the prostate permanently as they do in Brachytherapy. HDR therapy is almost always followed by 3D XRT for a shortened period and often preceded by a two-three month course of hormones. I didn't qualify, in his opinion, mostly because of the smallness of my tumor and it's particular location. Had it been at the extreme upper "base" of the prostate gland, he might have felt differently because the needles used in permanent seeding sometimes have trouble reaching up there, but since it wasn't and because of what he believed to be my generally positive prognosis he didn't believe his procedure to be appropriate for me.

He did, however, take time to explain each of the various treatment modalities presently available and to give me his opinion of each, considering my particular prognosis. He reiterated Mack Roach's view that it looked like the results from each of the major treatment modalities were all coming out the same. He explained that if you look at the comparables at eight years, (as far as we can go back because of the newness of some of the radiation disciplines), there's no difference in their efficacy. Radical Prostatectomy, 3D conformal radiation, proton radiation, high dose radiation and interstitial seeding (Brachytherapy) all appear to be viable options. Only standard external beam radiation and cryotherapy seem markedly inferior. I would add to this my own discovery that almost every physician in the American medical community believes that watchful waiting should be on the list of undesirable alternatives, though many knowledgeable and intelligent men choose it every day. If anything, I suspect it's becoming increasingly popular, out of frustration with the blur of confusion that greets so many newly diagnosed men. Since it doesn't interrupt your life and since the progress of most prostate cancers tends to be slow and the growth of a specific tumor is very difficult to predict, its potentially very attractive for men who prefer an alternative approach, especially when combined with something else like a non-fat diet, herbal or aroma therapy or intense nutritional supplement use.

While Mate felt that Brachytherapy was a serious option for me he said that if it were him, he'd probably go the surgery route in the end. As an MD, his assessment of the odds that my tumor was encapsulated was 85 - 90% so he believed surgery to be the most certain route available at the current time and that it would give me the greatest potential to live out my life expectancy. He recommended people to see in each treatment area, some of whom I already had visited, explained his view on the reported morbidity's (negative side effects) of each and then I was on my way. But, I was leaving with much greater balance and perspective and the information was coming openly and fairly from someone who had excluded himself from personal gain or involvement of any kind.

Blasko was even more painstakingly objective in his approach. He explained that he had only actually begun the modern version of seeding in 1987, and since he wasn't certain it would work or what the side effect profile might be, he had initially only treated men who were elderly or whose disease was quite advanced. As he got more comfortable with the procedure and as the data suggested enhanced success, he began using it on increasingly younger men until about four years ago when he started applying it freely to men of all ages when he deemed it appropriate. He was impeccably modest in answering my questions and in the explanation of what, why and how he does his thing. I would have to personally decide on what to do, without his influence. He was extremely complementary towards many of the people I had recently seen, particularly at UCSF, identifying them as some of the best in the country in their respective roles. Then, he carefully explained his view of the pivotal issues in making up one's mind about what to do.

First, I should try, with his and my other physician's help, to evaluate what kind of overall medical candidate I am. I should attempt to estimate the likelihood of the cancer being confined to my prostate, the size and location of my disease, my general health, etc. I must understand that there is always a possibility that the cancer has metastasized "microscopically" and there would be no way to detect it, but I couldn't let that possibility drive my decision. Then I should think about what side effect problems are likely to accompany each different treatment, considering the size of my prostate, any pre-existing problems with prostatitis or urethritis, my sexual history, etc. I should gauge each possibility in terms of whether it fits with my quality of life desires, my life expectancy concerns, the certainty of success, etc. Am I the type of person who has to believe that the cancer is gone from my body completely or can I live with the possibility that it is still inside me, though it may stay dormant and never again be a problem? Some men can't abide the notion that the disease is still inside their bodies, even if it may forever be quiet and non-destructive. They need to have it taken out and they want to see it in that proverbial bottle.

It was a good time to have this discussion, because I finally felt ready for it. I'd spent a lot of time and effort trying to determine why it was that so many men who had chosen surgery apparently needed follow-up radiation therapy or some other additional treatment. I had attempted to create real data on recurrences overall, either local (in the prostate gland itself) or distant (in another organ or structure) regardless of which approach one chose. While nobody seemed to have actual numbers, virtually every person I spoke to offered assurance that in his practice it wasn't likely or frequent. But I was becoming increasingly aware that this was a major issue for me and would become a critical factor in my final choice. I actually had been told by a physician I genuinely like and respect that a number of recent studies had shown recurrences 10 years after surgery running above 60%, as measured by whether or not the patient's PSA was detectable. This seems to be a pretty well kept secret. I couldn't believe the number was really that high so I arbitrarily brought it down to 50% overall to make it seem more reasonable. Still, it was incredible to me that so many men would consider submitting to the torture of this procedure if the probability of the disease returning is so significant.

Blasko insisted that there just wasn't enough data yet available to make exacting comparisons and therefore that younger men who wanted to go with better established precedent and a longer track record should not dismiss surgery. In fact, like Tim Mate, if it were his disease he might well choose that course over his own Brachytherapy or 3D conformal radiation because his medical school training and general scientific orientation would force him to seek the best known, most used and, by definition, most conventional approach available at the present time. He's changed his mind today because of more recent positive data, but that was his position at the time. It was certainly the conservative answer, though not necessarily the one I wanted to hear.

Nonetheless, however limited the data might be, here's what they were showing: Walsh's ten year overall results, presumably the highest standard of comparison, showed that 70% of his patients had zero or negligible PSA's. The comparable overall results for seeding, though only seven years worth, put 85% of the patients in that same minimal PSA category. But it was not impossible, Dr. Blasko stressed, that within that three year differential lay the possibility for the Brachytherapy numbers to come down enough to become even with the surgical results or to even possibly go slightly below them. There was just no way to know, but he believed an outcome of virtual equality to be a reasonable expectation. In all likelihood, "they would probably end up looking exactly the same".

As to the side effect profile, the evidence did seem to very strongly favor seeding over the other choices. Blasko's procedures had resulted in almost no incontinence. He had treated only one man who developed serious leakage and that gentleman had the misfortune of having pre-existing Parkinson's Disease. But on the negative side, I should remember that an inevitable consequence of permanent seeding was a number of months of much greater frequency and urgency of urination, especially for patients with larger prostates or men who had been exhibiting similar symptoms for some time prior to the seeding. Some small percentage of seeded men (about 10%) would need to wear catheters for awhile after the seeding. And, many of these side effects would not disappear completely for six to nine months after the procedure. As to rectal complications, there were considerably fewer than those produced by external beam radiation and, in his experience, they were so negligible as to be equal to surgical results in this specific morbidity. In fact, he had never had a patient with rectal fistulas or ulcers.

To properly assess the question of impotence, I must understand that no known treatment is particularly good news for erections, but seeding does seem to have the least negative impact and by quite a lot. The mechanism by which the seeds cause the injury that produces impotence is very different. In the case of surgery, one or both of the nerve bundles, are physically removed, rendering an erection either more difficult or almost physically impossible. Radiation's mischief comes from the scar tissue (fibrosis) that results from it's burn so that the effected tissue can surround and entrap the nerves and block them and other vessels that supply blood to the prostate. The degree and impact of scar tissue that actually forms seems to be a function of each individual's bodily reaction as well as the quality of the physician administering it. As with surgery, if the specifics of the patient's condition appear right for it, there is a "nerve sparing" alternative that should produce a better potency result, but in any event one of the inevitable results of seeding is that since the prostate gland gets effectively dried up, the amount of ejaculate produced is severely reduced or eliminated.

The impotency percentage of men who choose seeding, overall, regardless of age, seems to run about 25%, while in 3D XRT, it probably approaches 35%, based on my survey of physicians and patients. Impotency from surgery, however, Blasko thought was at least 50% or twice as high as in Brachytherapy, but I believe, that this statistic is consistently underreported and understated and is, of course, extremely influenced by operator competency. The more accomplished the surgeon, the better the result. However, my own impartial but certainly incomplete survey concluded that the overall number of men rendered impotent by radical Prostatectomy probably exceeds 70%, a truly awful result.

Dr. Blasko then wanted to make sure that I really understood the technique of seeding and how it differs from the external beam type of radiation. In my case he would use palladium 103 seeds because he thought they would be more effective and that the shorter duration (17 day half life vs. 60 day half life of iodine) makes a patient's recovery speedier than with iodine seeds. The seeds are placed on what amounts to bullets of titanium and then actually implanted into the prostate on needles that penetrate your perineum (the area below the scrotum), which will be both sore and discolored for weeks afterward The needles are guided into position by an ultrasound device which shows your prostate gland to the physicians well enough for them to seed the gland evenly and precisely.

The whole process would take a couple of hours at most, I could leave the hospital that afternoon, I probably wouldn't need a catheter and I could choose either a general or a local anesthetic. He'd need to see me the next day to check the results to see where the seeds had settled and to make sure that I felt all right and answer any additional questions. Then I could head home to San Francisco and when I felt ready, probably within a week or two, return to my normal schedule or some reasonable version thereof.

The seeds should get absorbed into the prostate very quickly and held there, but there is a measurable risk (less than 10%) that one or more could migrate to the lung or be passed through the bladder and out of my body. This was probably of no serious medical concern or consequence but that wasn't yet totally proven and in the interest of my fully understanding the whole process, he at least wanted me to be aware of it. There were a number of other details, but we could cover them at a later date should I choose to proceed. Finally, and to further complicate the process, I should know that if I took this route I could choose seeding alone or precede it either with external beam radiation or with a hormonal blockade or both. He explained each possibility at length but would not venture an opinion, at least until I had thought out and further investigated each one.

Dr. Blasko very humbly acknowledged the rather substantial increase in the recent popularity of the procedure. He promised me that, as in every case he accepts, he would do it himself if I ultimately chose to go ahead. He reminded me again of the sparseness of the data and assured me that I could and absolutely should take my time to decide. In fact, that was the only really strong opinion he offered on any subject during the entire hour and a half we had spent together.

"Be deliberate and don't rush into a decision. You'll need to feel happy with your choice for the rest of your life." He assured me that the probability of any serious change in my condition over the next couple of months was very low and any such danger was greatly outweighed by the negative consequences of feeling that I had rushed into a wrong decision.

Man-o-man did I feel better. I had been helped to lots of new information in the last week and I felt the freedom that goes along with it. I knew I still had a little more to do but I was getting the sense I desperately needed that the process wasn't infinite. I actually was going to be able to make my own "informed guess" and it had a reasonable chance of being the right one for me. Now I had to re-visit my notes, try to get greater perspective on the whole question and do some more research on the more subtle issues that had recently begun to emerge.

I had been monitoring the Internet for a while but after the last few interviews and some other conversations I had with patients, physicians and the CEO of the only company that was presently producing palladium seeds (Theragenics), I tuned in on the seed pods web site (http://rattler. cameron. edu/SeedPods). I read hundreds of communications from patients and a number of physicians which really helped me get a better sense of the pros and cons. Then I read a lot more of the literature that focused on recent data in seeding, both combined with other treatments and by itself, without any other conventional "adjunctive" therapies. And at the same time I stayed busy on the phone with other patients I had heard about through friends. It took less time to interview them because I had developed enough information and experience to know what to ask and how to hear their answers better. I had worked out a way to let men who had been operated on, externally radiated or permanently seeded tell me honestly how they were doing. Sometimes, by using an unspoken code, I could clearly understand their situation without embarrassing them or myself. Too high a percentage of the men I talked to volunteered their unhappiness with surgery and told me with great emotion that they thought they had made a big mistake by rushing into a decision, one which they wouldn't have made today, knowing more about the consequences and having heard about alternatives they really hadn't previously considered or even known about.

You have to feel in your inner soul that you've made the correct choice, after it's all done. For some men, such serenity might be found without doing anything other than seeing a single physician and immediately following his advice. While I'm skeptical about the quality of the information, maybe it's more important for them to be confident and happy going forward than to have chosen exactly the "right" procedure. If the prognosis is statistically about the same in any of the three major modalities, why all the fuss? For me and many other men whom I heard express themselves in meetings, personal dialogues on the Internet or in direct conversations, it wouldn't be possible to find happiness without looking the process in the eye and feeling our way through it. As one of the 'alternative' physicians I saw told me early on, "this is a decision of the heart, not the mind". But for me, my mind had to get my heart ready so that the inner peace so vital to success could ultimately be found.

I had taken a series of discrete steps which I now know I had to take, one at a time. I was very lucky to be able to afford to take the time necessary to accomplish them. First, I really had to try to figure out exactly what disease I had. As I've tried to explain, this is not a straightforward process. My pathologist, whom I had no role in selecting, botched the job miserably by understaging me, so my Gleason grading was wrong. Then he made matters worse by refusing to send my slides to the various physicians and laboratories who requested them because evidently he was too busy and he thought I was "shopping" my results. Remember, these are your slides to do with what you want; they belong to you and to no one else. Only when this jerk realized that I was serious about suing him did he cooperate. He's probably typical of many people who are "just doing their job" and consequently not paying enough attention to the patient or his welfare. But the point is that he really didn't know what he was doing and I and most of the people I was seeing were relying on his analysis to make a determination of what might ultimately happen to me.

I could have gone for yet another biopsy but I believe there is enough evidence to warn you away from doing this too often. While this procedure is often essential I feel it should only be performed when no other option exists, because of the possibility, however remote, that it may cause the release of microscopic cancer cells into the bloodstream. Use this test when you've reached the point at which there is no remaining choice, not as the first weapon when you begin to suspect the possibility of prostate cancer. Not only is it potentially dangerous, it's terribly inaccurate and primitive. There is a serious possibility of getting a "false negative" result. You can have successive biopsies and one will conclude you're normal while the next one definitively signals cancer. As in my own case, many men get the initial good news reversed as soon as the next biopsy is performed. There is no way to determine exactly where in the gland the core samples are actually coming from so the test is by definition only conclusive if it is positive; if it shows that you have cancer.

Only when you finally get confident that you have an accurate diagnosis, can you begin to decide how to handle the problem, what your choices are and which is best for you. In my case I began the process feeling completely overwhelmed. I didn't think I'd ever be able to find my way out of the maze. I learned to understand that the answer may be different for each of us. Each case is special and influenced by personal conditions and emotions. I just went with what finally felt most right to me. What else could I do? My decision certainly didn't come easily. I began with a strong preference for surgery and always assumed that I would end up there. But I became more and more skeptical as my search progressed. Maybe what turned me off was the attitude I encountered in many of the urologists I met. I don't like being talked down to and I don't trust people who treat me in a solicitous fashion. As a group, they were too complacent and self-satisfied for me and while that may not be good enough reason for the decision I made, I just couldn't get beyond it. If their way was so obviously the right one, why were so many of them didactic, defensive and unwilling to explore other avenues? Why weren't they better informed? I'm certainly not referring to all urologists, but the behavior I found objectionable I found to be the norm, not the exception.

Most importantly, when I got really objective about things and reached beyond my negative visceral reaction, I couldn't get past the question of why I should submit to such a major procedure with the potential for such enormously negative consequences if I couldn't be absolutely certain that it would work. The frequency of recurrence, a fact I really had to dig hard to uncover, completely removed the only important variable that would have made surgery the absolutely right choice for me. Fifty-fifty just wasn't good enough odds, I concluded, to take all the risks that inevitably accompany going under the knife.

External beam radiation, administered by one of two people I genuinely trusted and admired, both of whom are amongst the best in their field, was a very appealing possibility. But, in the end I wasn't as certain of its long-term efficacy as I needed to be and I couldn't get comfortable enough with the side-effect profile. I wouldn't be gaining that much potency benefit over surgery and the possibility of rectal complications, though readily dismissed by both men, kept getting reemphasized by every urologist I met. I got close, but it just didn't quite make it for me.

Watchful waiting really tempted me. My fellow participants in the Ornish program were all doing it and quite a few were showing some very early signs of possible progress. They were happy and their confidence was growing, so I was upset at the prospect of abandoning them. Right up until the day I left to have my procedure done I flirted with just staying the course and relying strictly on the program. After all, worldwide, there's a very large group of men who've opted to watch and wait, and whose outcomes, at least in the early years, are pretty much the same. I was taking lots of vitamin and nutritional supplements and feeling physically about as good as any time I could remember since my youth. In desperation, with only two days to go I reluctantly agreed to a deep meditation with Dean Ornish as my guide.

I went into it feeling it was much too "California" and generally too nutty for me. But I was in such emotional distress that I agreed to give it a try. After thanking my prostate for all the help it had given me over the years I asked it what to do. I learned that it was very tired from the battle it had recently been waging and losing. And, in the course of the next hour, it begged me, through very vivid imagery, to go get help. It could no longer handle the crisis alone and I should "bring on the cavalry" if necessary, to help fix the problem. While this was one of the first experiences of this type I had ever had and something I would not ordinarily do, the result was terrific. Ornish was startled and probably disappointed by the result but found it so conclusive that to his credit he strongly urged me to follow the advice. I emerged from the session startled by the clarity and decisiveness of the message and with renewed determination to go ahead.

The most positive choice for me and the one that made me feel most optimistic about my future was to have my prostate permanently implanted with radioactive seeds. After all my investigative research was finally over it emerged for me, personally, as the least invasive and best lifestyle choice. The physician I chose was someone I felt I could really trust. His approach, being very interested in my progress but unwilling to overtly influence my choice, felt right to me. It was only after I informed him of my decision to have Brachytherapy alone, without either a hormonal blockade or external beam radiation that he gave his opinion, one that I was delighted to hear: "For what it's worth, if it matters to you, your choice is exactly the one I'd have made in your exact circumstances." That reinforcement helped make the trauma of the previous four months feel worthwhile.

My procedure went smoothly and my physician described it to my waiting family as "boring", just how he hoped it would be. My five month recovery though difficult on a few occasions, generally went as comfortably as I had hoped. I'm fully functional and other than some early bouts with urgency and having to learn to plan ahead to be able to respond immediately to urges from my prostate, things have been relatively uneventful. I memorized where every accessible bathroom was located within a one mile radius of any place I regularly visited. I also became an expert on trees. It took me awhile to get the confidence to fly commercially, without intensely fearing a line for the lavatory. I had a recurring image of my knocking down innocent women and children in my urgency to get in there. But on balance, at least physically, it's been a piece of cake. I've had my moments of fear and depression but I think they would have occurred no matter what choice I made.

I have no idea if I made the correct decision or if such a thing actually exists, but I'm certain it was right for me and the best one I could have made. You have to go through it your own way and come to a conclusion based both on your physical circumstances and mostly how it all feels to you in the end. Remember your heart and you'll find genuine peace and comfort. An easy answer isn't achievable in a problem this complex but if you take control, open yourself to the people who care about you and proceed deliberately, with serious and optimistic determination to overcome the crisis, you have an excellent chance for a long and happy future.

FOOTNOTES

Johns Hopkins University
600 North Wolfe Street
Baltimore, Maryland 21287-8943
410/955-5000

University of California, San Francisco
400 Parnassus Avenue
San Francisco, California 94143-0330
415/476-8800

University of California, Los Angeles
School of Medicine
Urologic Oncology
10833 Le Conte, Room 66-118 CHS
Los Angeles, California 90095
310/206-1434

Loma Linda University Medical Center
Department of Radiation Medicine
11234 Anderson Street
Loma Linda, California 92354
909/824-4244

University of Texas
MD Anderson Cancer Center
1515 Holcombe Boulevard
Houston, Texas 77030-4095
713/792-8784

Northwestern University Medical School
Robert H. Lurie Cancer Center
Olson Pavilion
303 East Chicago Avenue
Chicago, Illinois 60611-3008
312/908-5250

University of Washington School of Medicine
University Cancer Center
University of Washington Medical Center
1959 Northeast Pacific Street
Box 356043
Seattle, Washington 98195
206/598-4100

University of Southern California
USC Comprehensive Cancer Center
Norris Hospital
1441 Eastlake Avenue
Los Angeles, California 90033
323/865-3900

Swedish Medical Center / First Hill
Tumor Institute
1221-1225 Madison Street
Seattle, Washington
1/800-422-4547

Memorial Sloan-Kettering Cancer Center
1275 York Avenue
New York, New York 10021
212/639-2000

The Mount Sinai Medical Center
5 East 98th Street
New York, New York 10029-6574
212/241-4812

Columbia Presbyterian Medical Center
212/305-2500

Seattle Prostate Institute
1101 Madison, Suite 1101
Seattle, Washington 98104
206/215-2480

The Preventive Medicine Research Institute
900 Bridgeway
Sausalito, California
415/332-2525

Christopher Logothetis, M.D.

Charles "Snuffy" Myers, M.D.

John Trachtenberg, M.D.

Howard Scher, M.D.

Eric Small, M.D.

Chapter 23

TAKING ON PROSTATE CANCER

by Andy Grove

Source: Fortune, May 13, 1996 v133 n9 p54(9).

Abstract: Intel's CEO recounts being diagnosed with prostate cancer and doing a great deal of research on the various types of treatment. He discusses surgery, radiation, cryosurgery and seeding and describes the high-dose radiation treatment he chose.

Text:

My secretary's face appeared in the conference room window. I could see from her look that it was the call I was expecting. I excused myself and bolted out of the room. When I stepped outside, she confirmed that my urologist was on the phone. I ran back to my office.

He came to the point immediately: "Andy, you have a tumor. It's mainly on the right side; there's a tiny bit on the left. It's a moderately aggressive one." Then, a bit of good news: "There are only slim odds that it has spread." The whole conversation was matter-of-fact, not a whole lot different than if we had been discussing lab results determining whether I had strep throat.

But what we were talking about was not strep throat. We were talking about prostate cancer.

Let me start at the beginning…

MY FIRST PSA. It all started about a year earlier when my family physician of 20 years retired. In the fall of 1994, my new physician gave me a physical exam to establish a new baseline. The physical involved an assortment of blood tests, all of which were in the normal range, with one exception. The test called PSA came back with a result of 5. The acceptable range, according to the lab computer, was 0 to 4.

I didn't know what this test was. In fact, I don't think I'd ever had one before. My physician's comment was, "It's slightly elevated. It's probably nothing to worry about, but I think you should see a urologist."

He did not seem too concerned, so I didn't get anxious, either. I put off the whole issue without much thought. I did, however, happen to tell one of my daughters, who is a health-care professional. She told a physician friend of hers, who, it so happens, was just publishing a long article on the pros and cons of screening people with this very same PSA test. Would I want to talk to him about it? I would. I did.

Oh, my God.

With that conversation, I parachuted into the middle of one of the raging controversies of contemporary medicine. Briefly, the issue, as I understood it, seemed to be this: A PSA test (PSA stands for prostate specific antigen) measures a substance emitted both by the normal prostate gland and by cancerous tissue in the prostate gland. Very little escapes from a healthy gland, so elevated PSA readings can be telltale signs of prostate cancer. But just because they can be doesn't mean that they always are.

Telling a person with an elevated PSA that he might have cancer leads him into a system of increasingly complex and uncomfortable diagnostic tests to ascertain whether it is so. If it is, the patient has to make some choices about what, if anything, to do. None of the choices, the friendly voice matter-of-factly explained to me on the phone, are good. None of the treatments work all the time, and all of them have side effects that are unpleasant or worse, like incontinence and impotence.

Anyway, according to my daughter's physician friend, prostate cancer isn't necessarily fatal. Autopsies show that about half of all men who die of other causes have some cancerous tissue in their prostate. So, my new acquaintance said, why submit unsuspecting men indiscriminately to this test, which only leads to more tests, which then lead to a series of choices, none of which are very good?

He sent me a preprint of his article. It was a scientific medical paper with charts, filled with learned discussion. But I picked up enough of the subtext so that my eagerness to visit a urologist, not very high to start with, waned some more.

It so happened that I was due to leave town on sabbatical in early 1995. I was planning to spend a month in the mountains skiing and writing a book. After a while, the PSA issue worked its way back to my consciousness. Having a computer with me and some time on my hands, I started looking for information on CompuServe. It wasn't hard to find. I found a prostate cancer forum where patients and relatives of patients swapped stories, asked questions of each other, and gave answers. The term PSA was mentioned in every message.

I also found a long review paper in the forum that was written by the head of the urology department at Stanford University, Dr. Thomas A. Stamey. I downloaded it, and I read it from beginning to end.

I found out some basic facts, such as: Some 200,000 men were diagnosed with prostate cancer in 1994, and 38,000 men were expected to die of it, making it the No. 2 cause of cancer deaths among men (after lung cancer). The paper discussed the seeming paradox of why such a small proportion of the people who have prostate cancer die of it, and speculated that most prostate cancer isn't very aggressive. I wondered, Is it not simply because most prostate cancer is diagnosed in older men who die of other diseases before the prostate cancer has a chance to get them? (This was not encouraging for me. I was only 58 and otherwise in perfect health. I couldn't wave the threat away with such an argument.)

Then the paper went through the treatment options. My daughter's friend was right. They were all lousy. The most prominent is surgical removal of the tumor. This is done by removing the whole prostate gland, then rebuilding the related internal organs. It's major surgery, with a long recovery and pretty bad side effects. Dr. Stamey's article only hinted at how unpleasant they are. I read a posting on the forum by an airline pilot who had undergone this surgery and was bitter beyond words. He claimed that it cost him his health, his job, and his marriage, and that it ruined his life. It was all very depressing.

But the important thing I took away from this essay was the concept that PSA is a tumor marker. It seemed that the larger the tumor, the higher the PSA. My own result of 5 seemed to correspond to a tumor the size of a sugar cube. I visualized a sugar-cube-sized tumor inside me, and I shuddered.

I came across a mention of a book on prostate cancer, jointly written by a patient and his physician. I ordered it and when I returned home after my sabbatical, I picked it up. It was quite readable, a thorough and organized review of different treatments, but it was noncommittal. The book itself reflected the contradictions of the literature, without providing guidance as to what course of treatment is best.

I went back and had a repeat PSA test done. As in my case we were looking at a difference in PSA readings of 4 (the upper range of acceptable) and 5, I wondered if the tests were precise enough. So I also decided to test the tests. I had my blood sent to two different labs. Unfortunately, what I hoped for—widely varying results—did not materialize. One test came back at 6.0, the other at 6.1. It appeared that the sugar cube was growing.

These tests ended my procrastination. I made an appointment with a urologist. He first checked my prostate with his finger (this test is called a digital rectal exam, or DRE), and he didn't feel anything. But given my PSA, he did a biopsy a week or so later (not a pleasant experience but not a terrible one either). The biopsy turned out to be positive. Hence the conversation that started with "Andy, you have a tumor."

R&D. I went back to see the urologist. He sat me down and told me my options: surgery, radiation, cryosurgery (in which the tumor is destroyed by freezing it), and, finally, doing nothing and playing the odds. This is euphemistically called "watchful waiting." He told me that in my case "surgery would have a reasonably good chance of getting rid of the tumor." He gave me the impression that the other treatments would have a lower probability of curing me.

He walked me through the complications of surgery, but reassured me: "Don't worry, we can do something about each of those." The examining room walls were covered with posters of contraptions like penile implants and vacuum pumps. I knew that they were devices meant to restore potency, but they evoked images of medieval torture.

I was sent to the hospital to undergo two complex tests. In the first, a bone scan, an instrument scanned my body looking for signs of metastasis—advanced prostate cancer tends to spread to the bones. The second was an MRI, a long and mildly uncomfortable procedure, which looks for evidence of spread into the abdomen. Both were negative, but I got the impression that neither test was all that sensitive, so there might very well be disease that they wouldn't pick up.

I wanted to know more. I called a number of friends who are physicians, who came back with names and phone numbers of prominent practitioners of the different types of treatment. I also decided to dust off my research background and go directly to the original literature. I wrote out the first batch of titles from the bibliography in the prostate cancer book I'd bought, and my wife got copies of these articles from Stanford. My life entered a new routine. By day, I set up appointments. This was a royal pain. The physicians were hard to get hold of, and when they called back, I was often in meetings, so making one appointment required half a dozen phone calls. By night, I read scientific papers, plotting and cross-plotting the data from one paper with the results from another. As I noted other interesting references from these papers, I would ask my wife to get them on her next trip to the library. This whole exercise reminded me of my younger days, when I did the same thing in the field of semiconductor devices.

Meanwhile, life went on. I had to concentrate on work, which turned out to be a good thing, because it meant I could think about cancer only while I was actually doing my R&D. What suffered was time for sleep. Fortunately, prostate cancer is completely asymptomatic for a long time; my energy level was as good as ever and I was able to keep up with the extra load.

At first, the papers were overwhelmingly confusing. But the more I read, the clearer they got, just as had been the case when I was studying silicon device physics 30 years ago. That added a strange element of enjoyment to a process that was, overall, very scary. I remember how creepy it felt the first time I walked through a hospital door labeled RADIATION ONCOLOGY.

The appointments led to more appointments, the papers led to more papers. A physician friend ran a computerized search on a number of researchers' names I gave him. From this search I got a bunch of papers that were written in the last six to nine months—written after my reference book was published, in other words. Some of these turned out to be the most significant ones in this whole exercise. The field was hopping, not just with new work and discoveries but with controversy.

Each medical specialty—surgery, cryosurgery, different branches of radiology—favored its own approach. I listened to the audiotape of a long interdisciplinary medical meeting called, appropriately enough, "Prostate Cancer Shootout." I could sense the undercurrents of strong disagreement, couched in polite, faux-respectful terms. I had the impression that the people whose comments I heard had made the exact same comments in meetings before this one and would make them again in the future. The tenors always sang tenor, the baritones, baritone, and the basses, bass. As a patient whose life and well-being depended on a meeting of minds, I realized I would have to do some cross-disciplinary work on my own.

WHAT I LEARNED. The most important thing I learned was that the use of the PSA test reset the entire field of prostate cancer studies. PSA tests went into use only about ten years ago. Their use moved everything forward in time Typically, a PSA test can indicate the presence of prostate cancer as much as five years earlier than diagnosis by other means, like digital rectal exam.

Not only does this allow for earlier treatment, but it also has an important consequence from a scientific standpoint: We can now learn a lot more about the effectiveness of various treatments by using the PSA test to look for recurrence of the disease. It used to take ten years or more for recurrences to be discovered by DRE and other clinical means. But since PSA can detect recurrence much earlier, the learning process about the effectiveness of treatment is accelerated.

Since the PSA test accelerates the discovery of the tumor in the first place, you have the chance to treat tumors earlier than ever before. One physician I met told me that all the treatments basically work quite well if you embark on them when your PSA is still relatively low. By contrast, none of them work well if it's high. Being a marker of tumor size, a high PSA suggests that the tumor is large, and a large tumor often extends outside the prostate gland to other parts of the body and can begin the process of metastasizing.

At this point I got a shock. I had an ultrasound imaging test done on my prostate to look for the shape and extent of the tumor. Most ultrasound machines give very ambiguous results, so much so that they are pretty much disregarded as diagnostic tools. But I had this done at a university hospital, where they have a very elaborate, newfangled machine that, in the hands of expert interpreters, supposedly gives more definitive results. In my case, the test suggested that there was a 60% chance that I had extracapsular extension, that is, the tumor extended outside of the prostate gland. I got depressed. Yet I soon found out that this should not have been a surprise at all.

Perhaps the most important paper I came across was a recent study by a group of physicians at Johns Hopkins looking at ten-year results after surgery on some 700 patients. In this study, they correlated the clinical findings—the medical findings on each patient before surgery, such as his PSA, the size of his tumor as established by digital rectal exam, and the biopsy results—with what the pathologists found during surgery. These results were then tabulated. The tables were extremely useful. They allowed me to look up any set of clinical findings and assess the statistical probability of the nature of the cancer in a minute. I had a PSA of 6, with the tumor largely contained in one half of the prostate and found by the biopsy to be moderately aggressive. When I looked up this set of clinical findings in the table, it showed that the chance of my having extracapsular extension was, in fact, about 60%.

The significance of this was contained in a companion paper, which correlated the chance of recurrence of the cancer with the medical observations before surgery. It found that even though the population of patients was carefully selected in terms of being good candidates for surgery, and even though all the operations were performed by one of the best prostate surgeons in the country, many of the patients experienced a recurrence of prostate cancer as indicated by their PSAs starting to rise again. When these patients were classified, the data showed that patients whose cancer was completely contained in the prostate gland experienced the lowest rate of recurrence, patients who had extracapsular extension experienced more frequent recurrence, and patients whose tumor had penetrated other organs near the prostate had an even greater chance of recurrence. I could see in these data what I had been told earlier: Surgery (like everything else) seems to work better at a low PSA.

In my case, if I didn't have any extracapsular extension, the data suggested that if I had a leading surgeon operate on me, I would have only a 15% chance of recurrence in ten years. If I did have extracapsular extension, I would have a 60% chance of recurrence at that time. And I had about a 60% chance of being in the latter class. Computing the odds based on these numbers suggested that my recurrence rate in ten years worked out to about 40%. I wasn't crazy about those odds. Clearly, surgery did not cure everyone, even under the best conditions.

Then there was the question of side effects. As indicated by the CompuServe posting from the airline pilot, these could be pretty bad after surgery. How bad depended on whose data I looked at. According to the surgeons who write papers, the side effects are not so bad. But I also read a study that questioned a large group of patients directly, and those results were alarming: The reports of incontinence and impotence were dramatically worse in the second study, leaving me to wonder whether patients described these things to a third party more pessimistically than to their physicians, or whether patients in the second study were more representative of the work and results of urologists all over the United States, as compared with leading practitioners. In any case, these certainly motivated me to examine other types of treatment.

Prime among these was external radiation. While surgery works by cutting out the tumor along with the rest of the prostate, radiation works by bombarding the area of the prostate, selectively causing more destruction of the cancerous cells than of the healthy ones. There's a lot of controversy about how well this works. Although there seems to be agreement that the side effects associated with radiation treatment are substantially less than with surgery, the effectiveness of the treatment is another issue.

It was especially difficult to get a good handle on the effectiveness of radiation because of the presumption by most urologists that surgery works best. Consequently, younger and healthier patients, particularly patients considered to be good candidates for surgery on account of their tumors being smaller, are selected for surgery, leaving the older, less healthy patients with more advanced tumors to make up the bulk of the patient population that undergoes radiation therapy. The results in the latter class are, of course, worse—reinforcing the spiral that sends the early-stage patients to surgery and the later-stage patients to radiation.

Yet in recent years, as enough patients with lower PSAs have overcome this selection bias and chosen radiation, data have emerged to show that results with radiation are also a lot better when the tumor is treated at an early stage. I came across a study that showed radiation therapy results and related them to the patient's initial PSA. When I took the radiation treatment data and compared them with the surgical data, matching the initial PSAs of the patient populations as best I could, the outcomes were not that different, at least at five years after treatment. (See chart on "recurrence rates.")

When I was doing semiconductor device research, it was expected that I would compare my results with other people's previously published results and that I would comment on any differences. But it seemed to be different in medicine. Medical practitioners primarily tended to publish their own data; they often didn't compare their data with the data of other practitioners, even in their own field, let alone with the results of other types of treatments for the same condition. So I kept on doing cross-comparisons as best I could.

I read about another radiation technique. Radiation can also be delivered to the prostate by implanting radioactive seeds directly into the gland. This was not a new idea. It was tried decades ago and discarded because the results were poor; it seems that the placement of the seeds wasn't uniform enough, leaving "cold spots" between them, and consequently the tumor wasn't completely eradicated.

More recently, however, this technique was being refined. Using ultrasound machines, the physicians could place the seeds far more uniformly and minimize the chances of cold spots. The seeds were left in the body, emitting radiation for six to nine months. The radiation would eventually decay, even though the seeds would stay in place indefinitely. Often the seed therapy (formally called Brachytherapy) was combined with external radiation just to ensure that the coverage was complete; even if the seeds should migrate around within the prostate, all parts of the tissue would get some radiation.

While I found references to Brachytherapy in my reference book, I could not find any good recent papers on it. I called the technical support department of the manufacturer of the radioactive seeds, and got quite a bit of information from them. The results, at least at five years, looked very good. The technical people also gave me the names of some of the practitioners of this technique. Then, in the middle of my search for information on this subject, a full paper was published that contained ten-year data on hundreds of patients who had been treated by a combination of seeds and external radiation. Unlike most, this paper actually compared the results with the best published surgical results. Basically, the two were very, very similar.

To make matters even more complicated, a physician friend faxed me an abstract of a presentation describing yet another procedure, a variant of the seed technique called high-dose-rate radiation. In this technique, a highly radioactive seed is attached to a wire that is momentarily inserted into the patient's prostate through a number of hollow tubes, one after the other. The procedure is performed with the patient under local anesthesia. The results in this abstract seemed even better than with regular seed therapy, especially when it came to side effects.

What particularly impressed me about both sets of data was that it seemed few of the recurrences were local, meaning that in the cases in which prostate cancer recurred, it usually didn't appear in the prostate but rather in some distant place in the body. This suggested that these combination radiation therapies are very effective in eradicating the tumor that's in the prostate. If the tumor had already escaped by the time the treatment was given, none of the therapies—not surgery, not any kind of radiation—could be expected to be effective.

The results looked good enough to warrant visits to two practitioners, both in Seattle. One practices seed therapy with the seeds left in; the other one practices high-dose-rate radiation with the seeds inserted for a short time and then removed. There was a logic to the high-dose-rate radiation therapy that really appealed to me. Evidently, one can compute how long the radioactive seed should stay in the prostate. The aim is to achieve a radiation exposure that is matched quite precisely to the size, shape, and location of the tumor. For instance, since the bulk of my tumor was on the right side of the prostate, the therapy could direct more radiation to the probable location of the tumor without having to expose the entire prostate to the higher levels of radiation. It's a programmable technique, customizable to seeds were more like carpet bombing. This was important because the side effects in the case of radiation come from exposing the neighboring organs, like the urethra and the rectum, to radiation. If one could irradiate the tumor heavily while minimizing the exposure of the other organs, theoretically one should get good results with minimal side effects. In fact, this was consistent with this physician's results. I sat in his office absorbing the elegance of this technique, and then I turned to him. "If you had what I have, what would you do?" He hesitated. Then he said, "I would probably have surgery." I left, utterly confused—but with some more unpublished data from the two seed physicians that I could add to my charts.

There was one more treatment to consider: cryosurgery. In this technique, instead of cutting the tumor out or blasting it with radiation, physicians freeze the tumor with little coils filled with liquid nitrogen that are inserted in the prostate under anesthesia. I couldn't find any hard data on the results of this technique, and it seemed that the side effects are almost as bad as they are with surgery. I took it out of the running.

I also found that a recent school of thought suggests that both radiation and surgical results can be improved by taking certain testosterone-suppressing hormones that cause the tumor to shrink. The shrunken tumor, I understand, is easier to cut out or to blast away. Since hormones seemed to help both surgery and radiation, I started taking them under the "smart bomb" physician's suggestion. The hormones had their own side effects, supposedly temporary. I had mild diarrhea and lost all interest in sex.

Meanwhile, I continued with visits to three more well-known surgeons. All were ferociously opposed to the combination radiation therapy, or any radiation therapy whatsoever. One, for instance, suggested the likelihood of a need for a colostomy (this scared me enormously). Another argued that none of these therapies result in zero PSA after treatment, as successful surgery does. This puzzled me. Since some PSA is generated by the prostate tissue itself and radiation does not destroy the prostate tissue, why shouldn't the patient end up with some PSA after treatment? The conversation got so heated that my question was never answered.

Looking for counterarguments, I called up the "smart bomb" radiation oncologist. To my surprise, he took a very evenhanded and unexcited position on the controversy, even as he debunked the specific issues raised. He had never seen a single case of colostomy, for example; he speculated that it may have happened in the very early cases when the rectum was overradiated. With the modern technique, he assured me, in all likelihood that can be avoided.

It sounded good, but I had one last question. "Why," I asked, "would you have surgery done to yourself then?" He thought about it. Finally, he said, "You know, all through medical training, they drummed into us that the gold standard for prostate cancer is surgery. I guess that still shapes my thinking."

I continued with my investigations. I talked to people who had gone through various procedures, including two who had undergone the "smart bomb" procedure. When it was all said and done, I had talked with more than 15 physicians and half a dozen patients. I began to get the same information. I plotted all the relevant data I could find (see "how the treatments compare" chart). It was clear that some cancers recur with the passage of time after all the treatments and that the range of variations for each treatment can be quite broad. It also appeared that whatever recurrences take place come on gradually and that the better the results were at five years, the better they would be at ten.

In any case, it was time for a decision.

DECISION. In July 1995, I went on a weeklong bike trip with my wife and some friends. Hours of biking are good to let your mind roam and put a helpful distance between all the mind-numbing data and yourself. I prepared a "balance sheet," first in my mind, then on paper. It looked like this:

Pro: surgery: —It's the gold standard: All these people believe it's the better answer. Can they all be wrong? —If the tumor is truly contained inside the prostate, it seems to work well.

Pro: seeds plus radiation: —Looks like fewer complications, such as impotence and incontinence. By most accounts it is also easier to go through. —If my tumor has spread outside the prostate, the radiation can perhaps still get it, as the external radiation covers an area that's larger than the prostate gland.

I looked at the sheet and concluded that if I knew that my tumor was entirely contained, I would go with surgery. On the other hand, if

I knew that it wasn't, I would go with the combination radiation. The data said I had about an even chance. I kept riding my bike.

One of the arguments that surgeons tended to make against radiation was that the long-term results—that is, anything longer than ten years—were not as good as in surgery. This wasn't obvious from the data. PSA has only been around for ten years, so as far as I was concerned, both surgery and radiation had relevant data only for ten years or less, and not very much even at ten years. But it occurred to me that if combination radiation, which looked better to me than external radiation by itself, only gave me ten years of freedom from disease, I could buy myself a ten-year reprieve relatively inexpensively, considering that it's a lot less onerous treatment. I have a rule in my business: To see what can happen in the next ten years, look at what has happened in the last ten years. PSA happened in the last ten years, and it is transforming the diagnosis and treatment of prostate cancer. Big things, I reasoned, could happen in the next ten years.

But this argument only worked if the combination radiation treatment gave results comparable to surgery in the first place. All the surgeons said it didn't. The radiologists shyly suggested that it did. I fell back on my data. I looked at my plots. The data said that the treatment results were the same—maybe even better for seeds.

I decided to bet on my own charts. Midway through the week, I confirmed my appointment for high-dose-rate radiation treatment a few weeks later.

TREATMENT. The "smart bomb" physician said it would help him target his weapons if I had a special MRI procedure done that was more sensitive than the one I had earlier. I lucked out. The university hospital that has this capability was also experimenting with a new technique, in which chemicals injected into the patient's blood interact with the magnetic field of the MRI machine to produce an image of the tumor as a group of red dots superimposed on the image of the prostate. I was awestruck by this technique. I could actually see where the tumor was and, to my relief, I saw no evidence of it being outside the capsule. It was about the size of a sugar cube. I made sure this film arrived at the Seattle physician's office before me.

Then I headed up to Seattle. I had to check into the hospital at 5:30 in the morning on a Tuesday. Monday was a very hectic day at work, which was wonderful: I didn't have a chance to think about Tuesday at all. But when I settled in on the late-evening flight, the workday behind me, no computers, no phones, the anxiety hit. Although my wife was with me, I didn't feel like talking.

The next morning, I got on the conveyer belt. It was no different than any outpatient procedure: questionnaires and a seemingly unending series of nurses asking very similar questions, taking my temperature, taking blood, on and on. Then, anesthesia. Although it was local anesthesia, it made me zonk out. By the end of the procedure, during which they inserted 16 hollow needles through my crotch into my prostate, I remembered very little of what happened. One incident that stood out involved the attending urologist (the procedure was jointly done by a radiation oncologist and a urologist, who was responsible for placing the hollow needles in the right positions). As I was coming out of my daze, the urologist showed me how he had watched the needle insertion through a fiber-optic cable threaded in my urethra. He described how he could see the needles advancing one after another toward his eyes, as it were. It was very strange.

I was wheeled into a CAT scanner, where they checked the placement of the needles one more time. I later saw the film of my body with the parallel needles in it; it reminded me of a porcupine. They proceeded to do the radiation analysis. Given the shape and size of my prostate, the tumor, and the placement of the needles, they needed to figure out how long the radioactive seed should take traversing in and out of each of the hollow needles. The special MRI came in handy here. The radiation planners were able to use the shape of my tumor as shown by the MRI as the basis for their calculations.

Two youngish guys did the calculations. They didn't look like physicians. They looked as if they could be designing chips at Intel. The calculations went on forever. Tongue in cheek, I asked, "What kind of computer are you using?" I was told, seriously, that they were using a 286, a product that we introduced 13 years earlier and stopped producing four years ago.

Over the next 48 hours, I was wheeled into the radiation room four different times. Each time, a robotic-looking contraption drove the radioactive seed through each of the tubes, one after the other. Then it was all over. They took the needles out. My delighted physician gave me a high-five and discharged me. The next day I flew home, and the following day I was back at work.

Altogether, I was out of work for three days. After that, for a couple of weeks, things were back to normal. Then the external radiation phase started. This follow-up radiation was done in 28 daily doses, each of which took no more than a few minutes but was a bit of a nuisance.

I showed up at a local hospital every workday morning at 7:30 A.M. I would undress, get radiated, put my clothes back on, and go to work. A week or so into this phase, just as they predicted, I started to get tired in the afternoon. I solved the problem by going home at 4 o'clock, instead of my usual 6:30 or 7 o'clock. I'd take a nap for an hour, wake up, turn on my home computer, and complete my workday at home.

Sometimes I would have a late-afternoon meeting. On those days I checked into a nearby hotel, took my hour's nap, and went back to work as good as new, albeit a bit sheepish about what people might think about my checking into a local hotel in the middle of the afternoon. If they only knew how harmless I was.

To my great annoyance, I gained weight, probably because I had to change my diet. I couldn't eat roughage because of all the bombarding my bowels were getting, so I ate more rich stuff. I gained three or four pounds in five weeks, quite a bit for me.

Then the 28 days were over. I was done. No more hormones, no more radiation, no more naps. In a week or two, I started eating vegetables again, started losing the weight I'd gained, and regained my normal energy. The latter was most important. Three weeks after the end of radiation, I was scheduled to give the keynote speech at Telecom 95 in Geneva, Switzerland. The preparations for the speech were demanding, and the speech itself was the most high-profile of my career. Between Telecom 95 and other activities, I spent two weeks traveling in Europe. All systems functioned just fine. Everything seemed to be back to normal.

Except not quite. Right after radiation ended, I had my PSA checked, the first in a lifelong series of such tests in which they look for recurrence. Even though the results were good, it was a reminder that at least emotionally, things would never be altogether "normal" again.

Half a year and three PSA tests have since passed. My life has been the same as before: my energy, well-being, physical functions (including sex). Still, periodically I have to face the dread of a PSA test. And although the results of the first three tests were very good, I know I will be stuck with this fear for the rest of my life.

SOME CONCLUSIONS. As a result of my progression through the experience of prostate cancer, I arrived at a few conclusions:

—First, tumors grow. Sometimes they grow quickly, sometimes very slowly, but they do grow. I think you should hit a tumor with what you believe is your best shot, early and hard. In my case, it was a combination of hormones, high-dose-rate implant radiation and external radiation. For others, like Senator Dole and General Schwarzkopf, it was surgery. If my best friend had this disease, my advice to him would be, "Investigate, choose, and do—and do save the best for later."

—All the debates notwithstanding, PSA tests are a godsend. They give you the next best thing to not having cancer: They give you time. I cannot comprehend the arguments reflected by my daughter's physician friend that we shouldn't do them because the treatment options aren't perfect. Using that same argument, should we not eliminate digital rectal exams? After all, both of them do the same thing: They signal the presence of prostate cancer. PSA just does it earlier.

I feel very strongly that if you are a middle-aged man, you should have this test done regularly; given the rapid rate at which some prostate cancers grow, I would opt for a frequency of once a year. You should know your PSA number just as you know your cholesterol count. Remember, it's a marker. What PSA gives you is the chance to act early. Don't blow it.

I shared what had happened to me and what I'd learned with a handful of friends and close associates. I learned that three of them had elevated PSAs. They were riddled with anxiety but hadn't done anything about it. I ran into another friend who had two relatives with prostate cancer, which greatly increases the likelihood of his getting it himself. Yet he hadn't had a PSA test. When I sit in meetings at work and look at groups of men who are my contemporaries, I want to shout at them, "Do you guys know what your PSA is?"

—There is no good gatekeeper in this business. Your general internist is not; the field of prostate cancer is a complex and changing specialty. Neither is a urologist; urologists have a natural preference toward surgery, perhaps because urologists are surgeons and surgery is what they know best. Any other treatment is deemed experimental even if it has just as much data associated with it. My review of the data led me to conclude that there are viable alternatives.

The whole thing reminds me of the uncomfortable feeling I experienced when I first sought out investment advice. After a while, it dawned on me that financial advisers, well intentioned and competent as they might have been, were all favoring their own financial instruments. I concluded that I had to undertake the generalist's job myself; I had to take the high-level management of my investments into my own hands. Similarly, given the structure of the medical practice associated with prostate cancer, that's the only viable choice any patient has. If you look after your investments, I think you should look after your life as well. Investigate things, come to your own conclusions, don't take any one recommendation as gospel. For starters, know where your case fits in the Johns Hopkins tables—this tells you volumes about your condition. In fact, I think these tables ought to be posted on the walls of every urologist's office. They should be viewed as the point of departure for a prostate cancer patient's bill of rights.

The right answer, in my view, can be arrived at only by comparing the results achieved by the practitioners of all the different treatment forms. This would best be done by cross-disciplinary work. Frankly, I am not impressed by what I encountered of this.

In the paper by Dr. Stamey, the one I downloaded from CompuServe at the outset of my odyssey, he says, "…when faced with a serious illness beyond our comprehension, [each of us] becomes childlike, afraid, and looking for someone to tell us what to do. It is an awesome responsibility for the surgeon to present the options to a patient with prostate cancer in such a way that he does not impose his prejudices which may or may not be based on the best objective information." I think we have a long way to go to reach this ideal.

WHAT WAS THE CHANCE THAT MY TUMOR EXTENDED BEYOND THE PROSTATE CAPSULE?

—In the course of surgery, physicians studied the actual nature of prostate tumors and correlated their findings to what urologists had observed during examinations before surgery. The results are tabulated in what I refer to as the Johns Hopkins tables.

This particular one shows the probability—expressed as a percentage—that the tumor penetrated the prostate capsule. The horizontal heading shows the size of the tumor (size increases left to right); the vertical numbers on the left, called the Gleason rate, indicate how aggressive the cancer cells are (the larger the number, the more aggressive the tumor).

In my case, some urologists said I had a T2a tumor; others characterized it as a T2b. My cancer cells had a Gleason score of 7. These numbers placed me in the green area, pointing to a 49% to 68% probability that my tumor went through the prostate capsule. I averaged those numbers and put my odds at 60%.

>From A.W. Partin and others, Johns Hopkins, Journal of Urology, Vol. 150, pp. 110-14, July 1993.

Johns Hopkins Table[*]

Percent of tumors penetrating prostate capsule

GROWTH

RATE
FASTER SIZE OF TUMOR LARGER

	T1a	T1b	T2a	T2b	T2c
2-4	0	22%	19%	34%	27%
5	0	29%	28%	45%	34%

* For patients with PSA between 4.1 and 10.0

6	0	45%	38%	56%	49%
7	0	58%	49%	68%	59%
8-10	0	64%	59%	77%	71%

WHAT WERE THE RECURRENCE RATES AFTER DIFFERENT TREATMENTS?

This was my first attempt to compare the results of different types of treatments. This chart shows the percentage of patients who experience rising PSA levels, the first sign of a possible recurrence of the disease, five years after treatment. I tried to look for data where the pretreatment PSAs were similar. In these cases, the patient populations predominantly had pretreatment PSAs below 20.

The red bars pertain to surgery; one is a series done at UCLA (U), the other a series done at Johns Hopkins (H). The blue bar shows the result of external radiation, done at M.D. Anderson Cancer Center (A). The gold bars show the results of combination radiation: Brachytherapy (seeds) plus external radiation. The first two gold bars show the results of treatment where the seeds are permanently left in the prostate; the third bar shows results of high-dose-rate radiation, where a radioactive seed is inserted and removed at a predetermined rate.

SURGERY

U	UCLA [see note] 1	31%
H	Johns Hopkins	20%

EXTERNAL RADIATION

A	M.D. Anderson Cancer Center	27%

SEED THERAPY PLUS EXTERNAL RADIATION
Seeds are permanently left in

G	Radiotherapy Clinics of Georgia	19%
N	Northwest Tumor Institute [see note] 2	20%

[SEED THERAPY PLUS EXTERNAL RADIATION]
Seeds are inserted and removed

S	Swedish Medical Center [see note] 2	14%

U: from Trapasso and others, UCLA, Journal of Urology, Vol. 152, pp. 1821-25, November 1994; H: Walsh and others, Johns Hopkins, same place, pp. 1831-36; A: Zagars, same place, pp. 1786-91; G: from Critz and others, Radiotherapy Clinics of Georgia, Cancer, Vol. 75, No. 9, May 1, 1995, pp. 2384-91; N: from Blasko and others, Northwest Tumor Institute, charts I received during my visit; S: from Mate and Gottesman, Swedish Medical Center Tumor Institute, abstract I received during my visit, subsequently presented at the Ninth International Brachytherapy Working Conference, Nice, France, December 1995.

1 Data for a subset of patients undergoing treatment since 1987 show a 20% recurrence rate after five years. 2 Data at six years.

How did all these treatments compare in the longer run? This chart shows rates of recurrence after different kinds of treatment. It does so by plotting the percentage of patients who exhibit rising PSA numbers as a function of time since treatment. In most cases, patients had an initial PSA of less than 20. Three data points represent patient populations with more advanced disease. In these cases, I mark the data point with a downward-directed arrow, reflecting my expectation that, if data were available for patients with PSA less than 20, the point would probably move downward. (Note that rising PSA after treatment does not mean that prostate cancer has actually recurred;

some studies indicate that metastatic disease follows rising PSA by five years or so.)

F: Fox Chase Cancer Center, Lee and others, Journal of Clinical Oncology, Vol. 13, February 1995, pp. 464-69; SU: Stanford University, Hancock and others, prepublication manuscript I received during my visit, subsequently published in Journal of Urology, October 1995, pp. 1412-17; K: data presented by Georgi Kovaks, University of Kiel, Germany, at the Ninth International Brachytherapy Working Conference, Nice, France, December 1995 (these data are with the seeds inserted and removed). [Chart not available—line graph comparing percent of patients with rising PSA levels after various treatments from 0 to 10 years after treatment!

— End —

Chapter 24

THE MOUNTAIN MAN GOES FOR CRYOSURGERY

I am 76 years old and still hold my private pilots license and per the FAA to maintain my license I am required to have a bi-annual physical to keep my license active, so in August 2003 when the physical was due and as my PSA had been ranging from 3.2 to 4.6 for about 8 years I ask the flight surgeon to also request a PSA.

Yes, I passed the flight physical with flying colors but my PSA had spiked from 3.3 to 10.8 in just 2 years but then went back down to 3.2 in a few weeks. I then requested a biopsy as a follow up and it came back with 2 of 12 needles positive at about 5% and both were in the right apex.

Now most think it kind of weird, but I never let a little thing like this upset me in the least. My way of life is and always has been "NEVER WORRY and NEVER HURRY".

You see I feel that any problem large or small is just a situation that a needs a little attention or in other words, "LETS GET IT FIXED SO WE CAN GO ON DOWN THE ROAD".

The Urologist, Dr. Crouch that comes to our area from Cedar City, Utah about every 3 or 4 weeks did the biopsy and he suggested HDR as mono therapy and set up an appointment with Dr. Hayes at Gama West at the Salt Lake Regional Hospital, Salt Lake City.

Well after getting the results of the biopsy I had decided I was going to get it fixed and that is exactly what I intended to do.

As I had been researching different procedures, their results, after and side effects for a while as with the way my PSA had been running

I felt that some day something would have to be done. But I was really in no hurry.

Anyway I really didn't see any urgency, but I did go the 300 miles to Salt Lake City (which is the nearest place I could get professional prostate cancer advice), to see Dr. Hayes.

He is a very interesting person and appears to be quite knowledgeable and concerned about his patients. But after our about ninety minute visit I just was not that comfortable with the procedure and possible after and side effects.

I then set up an appointment with Dr. Sause at the LDS Hospital Radiology Department also in Salt Lake City for about 3 weeks later. We also had a long discussion, probably about 2 hours, and he did a volume study and a PSA that came back at 3.8. He said that the prostate volume was 30cc which although a bit larger than normal was well within Permanent Seeds range. He suggested permanent seeds also as mono therapy.

I even set up a tentative appointment for January 05, 2004 but after more research and the reading of all I could find on both of the main seeding related sites on the net, I just did not like what I read. So I canceled the appointment.

During my research I had read several quite positive reports on the Cryotherapy being done by Dr. Douglas Chinn, who, by the way is a second generation Urologist whose father has been in the forefront in Cryotherapy for many years. I decided to either call or email as many of his patients as I could find, to get feedback on Cryotherapy treatment and the results, and specifically after and side effects.

Finding that the results were about what I felt I could live with, while living over 45 miles from the nearest medical clinic and still run the ranch alone, I decided to call Dr. Chinn for a consult, which I did. He sent me quite a bit of real interesting information on Cryotherapy which I studied. He also told me that he has been doing Cryotherapy for over 10 years at about 100 patients a year.

I also researched all the latest equipment that is now being used for Cryotherapy including the fact that they use the same rectal ultrasound to set the Cryo Probes as they use to map for seeding or to place the radiation needles for HDR.

I also studied the warming catheters that they use to circulate warmed fluid through the penis, urethra and bladder to help prevent any of the old problems they had with Cryotherapy of freezing the urethra and rectum. The rectal ultrasound also helps keep the rectum from freezing.

Last but not least I studied how they use the thermocouples and how their use can make certain that they only freeze exactly what tissue they want to freeze and nothing else. All this made a real impression on me.

I set up an appointment with Dr. Chinn for 16:00 on November 19, 2003 and asked him to set a tentative schedule for me to have Cryotherapy the next day which was November 20, 2003.

As my wife is quite handicapped and should not be left alone overnight, I hired a lady to take care of her and a local teen age boy to watch things here on the ranch for me. I had decided that I could be back in about 2 days and that everything here would be fine for that long.

As it is only about 560 miles to Dr. Chinn's office and about 20 more to the hospital he uses I decided I could leave here about 07:30 and make it in plenty of time for the appointment. I didn't get out until about 08:00 but made it on time for the appointment, but was not as early as I wanted to be.

Dr. Chinn and I had a good meeting and I received a complete physical. Then he said that everything was set up for the next day, November 20, 2003 and I told him I would be there.

At 06:00 the next morning, November 20 I checked into the hospital and was in surgery at 08:00 with a spinal. I had decided on a spinal so I could watch what was going on and also so I wouldn't be groggy going home the next day.

Anyway, I watched on monitors as the probes and thermocouples were inserted, and then watched as the temperature came down then slowly went back up to thaw the tissue. He did this 3 times, it was all quite interesting.

I was taken to recovery at about 11:30, where I stayed until 12:30, when I got good movement back in my legs. Then I was taken back to my room with a folly catheter and I also had a suprapubic catheter inserted directly into the bladder through the lower abdomen just above the pubic hair line.

The folly was hooked to an irrigation bag and the suprapubic catheter was hooked to a drain bag. They had the irrigation line set at about 200cc per hour and back flushed the bladder overnight. I was allowed to get out of bed, but was tethered to the drain bag.

The next morning November 21 at about 07:30 the folly was pulled and the suprapubic was hooked to a leg bag.

At about 10:00 Dr. Chinn and another Dr. came in and looked at the leg bag and I was discharged. I told Dr. Chinn I was going to drive home alone that day (about 580 miles)

He said "I don't think it can be done" and I told him "Well, I bet we will find out today, won't we". Then I walked down to the admitting office and collected my belongings then walked about a block to my car and left.

It was about 11:00 when I pulled out of the parking lot. I had fueled just before I checked in, so I had enough gas to make it to Barstow CA., but I had to find a station there that had a full service pump.

Then I stopped in Las Vegas for lunch at an Arbys drive through and another full service station for fuel. I just didn't feel like getting out of the car with the leg bag hung on the way the hospital did it. And yes, I did stop along the road 4 times to empty the leg bag out the door. I got home about 19:45 and was quite tired, but I had absolutely no problem, not even any pain or very little discomfort on the way home.

I had a good night but woke up with quite a bit of swelling and discoloration in the scrotum area, but not much discomfort. I had been advised that unless I kept ice packs on that area most of the time for a week or two I would have to expect swelling and even discoloration.

On the way home I didn't have any ice or ice packs so guess I asked for it. Also I didn't use an ice pack except in the evening the rest of the time and the swelling and discoloration didn't go away for about a week and a half

The next morning, about 07:00, when I went out to feed my stock I found the teen-aged boy hadn't loaded the hay trailer as he was supposed to, so as usual I had to do it myself.

This is when I found out how much I use my belly to handle hay. I got it loaded and fed the penned cattle, and then went out and broke ice on water tanks and ponds. I then ran a check on some fences. I was only gone about an hour and a half, but was a bit tired when I got home.

While I was tired, I had no pain and very little discomfort, which mostly came from the suprapubic catheter sticking out my abdomen. It really was more of a bother than anything else, and always in the way, and it was to stay in for at least 4 to 6 weeks. Some have it in up to 9 weeks. I DON'T THINK SO!!!

Well, about 5 days later, I somehow got the tube twisted or kinked and it didn't drain. After about 3 or so hours I had to PEEEEE BAAAAD but the instructions were not to even try to pee for at least 2 weeks. Hey, if you got to go, you got to go. Then I found that the leg bag was completely empty.

That's when I started leaving the valve at the leg bag closed all the time just opening it to check for retention. Having none, I called Dr. Chinn and told him what had happened and that I wanted it out.

He said we could try it, but that it may need to go back in. Well, I made an appointment with the only surgeon within about 265 miles and had him call Dr. Chinn for him to tell the surgeon how he wanted it taken out.

I went in on December 01 and had the surgeon removed it. Everything has been perfect since.

I had my 90 day PSA about February 18, 2004 and it came back at <0.1 which they tell me is undetectable. Yes, I feel good about and so far and at about 130 days the only after or side effects I have had was that bit of swelling and minor urinary urgency for about 2 ½ to 3 weeks after the suprapubic catheter was removed. I did have to get up about 3 times a night for about 3 weeks after it was removed.

So far I have taken absolutely NO medication and have had absolutely no other side effects. And yes at 76 I am still potent, though not as often as a few years ago. I'm a bit disappointed as there is about no ejaculation, but I guess at this stage in my life I can live with that. With no prostate I guess there is nothing to make fluid.

Now my advice to anyone is as follows: First and foremost get more than one opinion. Then do your research and don't let anyone rush you. Find a procedure that you are comfortable with. Then find a doctor that you are completely comfortable with. Then, and only then, GET IT FIXED.

If you don't feel good about something get it explained. If you are still not comfortable with it do more research and discuss it with someone that you feel good with. After all that GET IT FIXED and don't look back.

Above all: NEVER WORRY and NEVER HURRY. Always remember that if WORRY ever sneaks in, LOGIC, for sure, won't stay around long.

The MtnMan high in the mountains in Nevada.

mtnman@idsely.com

Chapter 25

THE GUARDIAN ANGEL

Arlen O'Hara

When my husband, Mike, announced in October 1999 that his PSA had more than doubled in a year's time frame and it had been recommended that he have a biopsy to see if he had prostate cancer (PC), I was not too concerned. Mike was in very good shape for a 67 year old man. He had good eating habits and was very athletic. Imagine my shock when he announced that he had "flunked" the biopsy and had prostate cancer. The pamphlet that was sent home with him from the HMO described two possible treatments. One was surgery with a three week catheterization and the possible side effect of impotence and incontinence. The second was external radiation with the possible side effects of impotence, bladder injury, diarrhea and burning of the rectum. There was one paragraph which mentioned Brachytherapy or "seeds", but indicated that it was fairly new. The publishing date on this text read 1995, which was at least four years old. There had to be more up to date information on prostate cancer and treatments. We started our odyssey with visits to physicians, books on the subject, and information on the Internet.

Yellow note pads in hand, in addition to the physicians Mike met with alone, we met with two surgeons, three radiological oncologists, one Hormone Therapy Oncologist/Consultant, and one High Dose Rate Implant Radiation/IMRT External Radiation Specialist. What did we learn?

Because of the PSA test, physicians are finding lots of early Prostate Cancers which are treatable with a variety of options. Unfortunately there is no test to see which of these cancers will be aggressive and which will be slow growing, so some kind of action is necessary. Technology is moving at such a rapid rate that new treatments are being discovered all the time.

We learned that 3D Conformal External Radiation is only 6 years old and has had very good results, yet it may become antiquated by the newer IMRT (Peacock) External Radiation. To a man, all of the physicians said there was no rush and for Mike to take his time in making <u>his</u> decision. There is a lot of information out there. Some of it is contradictory and confusing. Many of the issues to consider when choosing treatment are judgment calls. They require familiarity with general concepts. Ask each physician how he feels about bone scans and Endo-rectal MRI's and you will get several different opinions. Learn about PSA's, Gleason scores and The Partin Tables. <u>There are no dumb questions</u>. This is your life you're dealing with. Remember, the physicians are employed by you and work for you. The <u>best</u> treatment does not exist. Put blinders on. <u>There is no right answer</u>. Choose the treatment that is <u>right for you</u>. Consider all the facts and then trust your gut feeling above all others. Make your decision.

Once you have chosen that treatment don't second guess yourself. Make sure that you choose a "star" physician with the best equipment. We found out that 90% of the external radiation treatment centers use standard radiation instead of the cutting edge 3D Conformal, IMRT or Proton because of the cost involved in buying the equipment. Just "any old guy" won't do. <u>If you have Medicare, consider yourself lucky. It is the Gold Card for the best medical treatment available.</u> If you can't use the physician and hospital that you want, explore other health care options. Mike was able to leave his HMO and go back to Medicare with supplemental coverage that allowed him to choose any physician and hospital in the U.S. with no pre-existing conditions!

Mike was in the intermediate risk category because his PSA was under 10 and his Gleason at a 6. <u>All</u> of the treatments were options for him;

1. Watchful Waiting (not advised because of the rapid jump in his PSA).
2. Radical Prostatectomy
3. External Radiation (which includes, Standard Radiation (used by 90% of the treatment centers), 3D Conformal External Radiation, IMRT External Radiation (The Peacock) and Proton Radiation done at Loma Linda Hospital.
4. Internal Radiation-Long term radiation called Brachytherapy or "seeds" and short term radiation which is called High Dose Rate Implant Radiation.
5. Cryosurgery-freezing
6. Hormone Therapy (usually used to shrink the prostate in preparation for a treatment option or when the cancer has spread).

Improve your diet. Cut out fat and red meat. Find out what foods are good for the prostate, such as cooked tomato products. Use soy milk if possible. Try Edamame Soy Beans for snacks. They are in the grocers' vegetable sections ready to eat and also come frozen ready for cooking. Experiment in cooking with tofu and soy products. They are in all the markets. I make great enchiladas with soy "meat" and soy cheese. These products taste terrible individually, but when combined with lots of other ingredients and flavors, they become very tasty. Tofu stir-fry is quite good with some added chicken strips. You can make great French Fries in the oven! Almost any dish can be duplicated with experimentation. Fortunately, Mike is not a finicky eater and was open to my experimentation's. With a little creativity, you can fool even yourself.

Remember to laugh at life. Mike and I had some good laughs as we went from physician to physician. We called ourselves "The Yellow Pad People" and always liked best the physician we talked to last! Exercise. Mike is a fiendish athlete, but if you are not into sports, walking is great. It can be done anytime and any place and it's a great way to explore all kinds of new neighborhoods!

The good news, as said to Mike by one of the physicians, is you probably will not die of prostate cancer, but of something else. This is not a hopeless situation. In 1993 Michael Milken, age 46, was diagnosed with PC after a biopsy was done when his PSA, during a routine exam, was shown to be 24!! When they found that it had affected his lymph nodes, his options for treatment were significantly reduced. He had hormone therapy and 3D Conformal Radiation, which was brand new, and his PSA dropped from 24 to O where it is today, seven years later.

Arlen's Suggested reading;

1. Prostate Cancer
   A Non-Surgical Perspective
   by Kent Wallner, M.D.
   Published by Smartmedicine Press
   Copyright April, 2000

2. The ABC's of Prostate Cancer
   by Joseph Oesterling, M.D. and Mark A. Moyad, M.P.H.
   Published by Madison Books
   Copyright 1997

3. The article by Willie Wienstein in this book

4. The Prostate Cancer Protection Plan
   The Foods, Supplements, and Drugs That Could Save Your Life
   by Dr. Bob Arnot
   Published by *Library of Congress Cataloging-in-Publication Data*
   Copyright 2000

5. The Taste for Living Cookbook
   Mike Milken's Favorite Recipes for Fighting Cancer
   by Beth Ginsberg and Mike Milken
   Produced by Allen & Osborne Inc.
   Copyright 1998

Chapter 26

HOPE FOR THE FUTURE

Michael O'Hara

The approach to these vital subjects are individual by nature. Any problems you have should be immediately customized by your specific medical statistics. In order to maximize the result, regarding prostate cancer, no one should be allowed to make the decision for you concerning the treatment to use - not your physician nor those doctors from which you seek a second and third opinion. Even your spouse or other family member should not be delegated the responsibility of making these types of potentially life and death judgments. Only you should ultimately make these crucial decisions.

There is a case to be considered for the position put forth by my fellow collaborators, Tom Alexander - Chapter 15, and Dr. Al Barrios - Chapter 16. They espouse the international and especially European view that a prostate cancer patient can avoid all invasive treatments and magnify his natural curative powers to eliminate the problem. In many countries the physicians do not even recommend to their patients that they have an annual PSA test.

The only difficulty I have with that approach is that no one really knows how fast growing each condition is. The ability to discern whether your prostate cancer cells will be active (virulent) and spread outside the prostate shell, or passive and stay put, is unclear. Thus far, the U.S. Federal Government has not taken this disease seriously enough to allocate sufficient funds to find that answer or the cure for prostate cancer disease. When queried, government representatives concur, but blame the male population for not being willing to vigorously come forth and make such a demand! This is the demand that I would like to see made in an increasingly strong and persuasive manner.

However, as Dr. Stan Brosman has informed us, the prostatectomy surgery techniques have measurably improved, and become less invasive. Secretary of State Colin Powell recently chose to follow his former military comrade, General Swartskoff in dealing with what has always been the "gold standard", most popular weapon of choice – surgery. The second most popular is the seeds, or brachytherapy. Ultrasound technology currently allow teams of specialists to implant the radioactive tiny seeds with far greater precision then in past decades. As the result of 14 years of affirmative data, the seeds procedure yield success comparative to the results of surgery, but with less invasive residue. Thus, this treatment is gaining quickly in popularity. While in 1992, just 2% of radiation therapy used seeds, the percentage is close to 40%. Some experts predict that that procedure will soon become number one for less advanced forms of Prostate Cancer, especially for men over fifty.

Evidence now indicates that a man whose cancer hasn't spread beyond the prostate stands a 90% chance of being disease-free after five years if he undergoes brachytherapy, traditional radiation or surgery. The external beam radiation treatments continue to take the longest amount of time, "on the table", with daily visits to a clinic for eight to ten weeks.

Let me review some of the principal elements worthy of consideration concerning your crucial prostate cancer treatment decision.

1. When analyzing your options, look past the first "sales" presentation made by your urologist/surgeon.
2. Get second opinions, and thirds and fourths, on each important element, especially your treatment options, in your decision making process.
3. Develop an action plan that starts with securing a second opinion on your prostate biopsy slides from Dr. John Epstein at Johns Hopkins in Baltimore.

4. Locate and meet early with the premier local oncologist to help you identify the best three or four specialists for the various prostate cancer treatments. Also secure his advice as to how much time you have to accomplish your research.
5. Use your oncologists name, and every business and social contact you can muster, in order to secure early appointments with the superstar physicians for each treatment, both regionally and nationally.
6. Arm yourself with all of your records and medical statistics so you can incorporate these into your personal sales pitch, first to secure appointments and then to interest those physicians you meet with and motivate them to invite you to become their patient. (Note: the more outstanding the prestige of the physician the more he will be qualifying you while you qualify him.)
7. Request an immediate written evaluation report from each physician you meet with so that you can use the best report as part of the marketing of your candidacy to each physician.
8. Arm yourself with a series of probing, aggressive questions to help you in the decision about treatment and in turn to determine the optimum specialist for you.
9. Develop an action plan and incorporate it into a PERT Chart or other time table framework that will cover each essential action that you will take and mold the timing of each action sequentially.
10. Develop a decision making formula that will both help you objectively evaluate all of your options, and then aid in making that optimum decision.
11. Develop a decision making process, utilizing the right affirmation to enable your psychological and spiritual powers to support you. This process will help you focus all of your efforts and energy on this major decision in your life by giving it the priority that it deserves.

12. Identify the optimum diet for you (soy products, tofu, colorful vegetables, grains) and use it with imagination energy and enthusiasm.
13. Select not only the best physician in the world in the treatment discipline that you choose from among the top physicians that you interview, but also the one that has the newest and best equipment.
14. Develop your habit patterns, with the help of your spouse or woman friend, so that you eat right, exercise right and think right in order to optimize your prospects for long term health and longevity.
15. While it is fresh in your mind, write down your experience, complete with both your success and failure elements as you went about flattening your learning curve, so that you will be in a position to assist the next friend or family member who has to go through the same ordeal.

Once you have done all your research and finally have made your decision, you can expect to be tested. I was by my son Ryan, whose opinion I respect and whom I love dearly. He asked me "Dad, are you sure you're not taking the easiest way out? It seems like you are selecting the least invasive treatment because of the reduced amount of side affects, thereby increasing your chances of dying." It is vital for you to anticipate and be able to strongly defend your position on such penetrating questions in a way that is best for both of you. My response was "thank you for your concern for my health and longevity. I assure you that I am not missing the forest by concentrating on the trees. I have researched this subject carefully and I have concluded that even though I am an excellent candidate for all of the procedures, the Seeds deliver several key elements for me that are as good or better than the more invasive procedures. At the same time the risk of more invasive treatments that could be life threatening have been eliminated and the recovery from the treatment will be considerably shorter. Basically it's a win-win situation for me, and your Mother, who has attended many of my research sessions totally agrees with my decision." At that point in this sensitive discussion I carefully led him through my decision making system outlined in Chapter Two step by step.

By doing the right kind of research you can deal with any question on this subject because you have used answering those questions as a tool to making your personal decision. Therefore, you are in a position of being able to firmly defend your decision with confidence and vigor. For you to maximize your defense against "The Big C" you must employ strong psychological warfare techniques. That way your body will follow your mentally affirmative lead and do its part in winning this ultimate victory.

A number of good things have come from my experience with prostate cancer.

1. My relationship with family and friends has become closer and more cherished than ever before.
2. I have never eaten better and healthier in my entire life.
3. I've invested time and money into other preventative medical procedures such as heart testing, colonoscopy, orthopedic soles, acid bath of forehead, skin care, GI Series, etc.
4. I appreciate and relish each day of my life much more.

It is my considered opinion that this prostate cancer message needs to be brought out of the closet and be strongly illuminated. It is hard for many in the medical profession to expose this subject with total accuracy, because some of the facts reflect poorly on some of their medical brotherhood. The very thought of physicians portrayed as salespeople - pitching a potential client for life, is one that most medical associations and individual physicians abhor. The combination of bias on the part of physicians and the desire for males with prostate cancer to keep quiet about their sensitive condition to the point even to fabricating the truth about their recovery statistics, has created a path of progress leading to the defeat of this prolific condition that is slow and winding. Since men put little pressure on

Federal agencies to help fight cancers, prostate cancer receives approximately one tenth of the research funds devoted to breast cancer and reportedly one percent of the moneys directed toward the cure for AIDS.

It is late 2004, and the National Cancer Institute has just announced their estimates for this year. The good news is that deaths from carcinoma of the prostate is down, but to 30,000. Thanks a lot, PSA early warning system, but that's still ten times the number of deaths from the 9/11 disaster. The bad news is that 211,000 news cases of prostate cancer have been reported. One fifth of American men will have this dread disease, and over one fifth will suffer, many times even more, from other problems of the prostate. Thanks a lot, fast foods and heredity.

Since my deep plunge into prevention, I have found a "cocktail" of vitamins that appear to be far superior to the mixture I have been imbibing for the past decade. It has even been possible to strongly improve on my immune system measurement, which will help me fight off the next disease that steps up to my plate!

I have past the four year anniversary of my 138 iodine seed prostate implementation. I am delighted to report that my essential "plumbing" - both elimination processes, and erection capability, remain in good working order. My PSA remains at a static and safe sub 1.0 level during the entire period.

I am convinced at this point that selecting Dr. Peter Grimm, from the Seattle Prostate Institute, the best physician with that specialty in the world with the best equipment, was the right decision for my prostate oriented statistics and my physiological views. I've never felt better, nor savored life more, than I do right now. My improved eating habits have me at my college volleyball playing weight, 185 pounds vs. my previous of 192-195 pound level.

In retrospect, the only thing that would have made my road less pressured and the specific decision making process smoother would have been to have had immediate access to a book on prostate cancer like this one. Then, when first appraised by my HMO physician that I had flunked my prostate biopsy, I would have been prepared to deal with the dilemma with a great deal less stress and frustration. Doing the vigorous research also placed my mind in position to instruct my body that the right kind of help was on the way, leading to an affirmative result, which is the best way to deal with these types of challenges.

It also sends the right message to our sons and daughters, setting the best possible example, day by day, of how to deal with difficult problems. The finest wish we could have for our children and grandchildren is that each will reach his or her potential, in whatever field they choose to plow. Each one needs to see the importance of getting and staying healthy, and when they are young, we can be their mirror.

I believe that it is fair to compare the preparation for the prevention and treatment decisions concerning prostate cancer with the preparation for competing in serious sport. Success in both command that we keep the health of our mind and body at an optimum level. Achieving the ability to stay healthy past the age of ninety is of much more value, in the long run, than the winning of any Gold Medal!

As my speeches on this subject have extended nationally and now internationally, I have discovered a huge void. Too few are motivating men to do the right thing regarding the prevention of prostate cancer, and no one is motivating our government to help with the funding of research to finally be able to identify the virulent prostate cancer cells that will kill many of us if we do not take the appropriate action.

The expansion of this second book into vital areas such as preventative measures and cures of prostate problems, in addition to cancer, has been very fruitful. I sincerely believe that it will prove to be rewarding for this now vastly expanded group of males, that are being given new, important information. It also touches the even greater pool of daughters, sisters and spouses for all those additional males.

While there is currently no one "silver bullet" that works for all, there are some rainbows contained in these pages. Due to my recent affiliation with PCRI (Prostate Cancer Research Institute), whose national mandate is to educate the male population, great energy and enthusiasm has been generated. There is an opportunity for you to be a part of this national effort. We would, therefore, invite you to join us in this battle against cancer. Any funds donated by you and/or other motivated friends, would be tax deductible, if made out to "PCRI - O'Hara Prostate Cancer Fund" (501C3) and sent to their headquarters at 5777 W. Century Blvd., Suite 885, L.A., Ca. 90045. PCRI then supplies the direct expenses to transport me nationally for presentations, interviews with written and electronic media, lobbying of the federal government (and AARP) to better support our cause, saving more male lives or just their quality of life. As our population ages, this cause becomes even more just! If you would like to discuss this subject further, please call me at 310 454-4547 (oharaent@aol.com) or PCRI Executive Director Glenn Weaver at 310 710-3510 (gdw@pcri.org).

Internationally, both Rotary International and the International Olympic Committee have agreed to meet with me in Athens this summer, to determine whether they can combine forces to support this vital cause. Rotary was instrumental in defeating polio around the world, in the past decade. For the past three years I have been trying to motivate them to come through for their own 1.2 million members, in every city and town throughout the world. Both organizations have similar demographics, predominately male, average age late 50's, which is the same age neighborhood for prostate cancer. These two strong organizations are extremely talented, have big hearts, and are totally committed to accomplishing great deeds for all of the world's peoples, one through service in every community, and the other through world sport. Please come together with us for this vital battle.

All of my fellow case study suppliers and talented prostate cancer physicians have joined me, by contributing their input for the above purposes. I feel extremely strong about completing this compendium of special knowledge concerning this vital subject, and hope that it will present you with an early and important tool, both for preventative reasons, and should you have the sudden "need to know", concerning treatment decisions. Their contact information, along with my own, is supplied below, for any follow up questions that you may have. Good hunting, and remember, when you stop learning, you start dying. Please continue to stay informed!

O'HARA POSTSCRIPT

It is March, 2004, and I have hit the four year anniversary of my 138 iodine seed prostate implementation. I am delighted to report that my essential "plumbing" - both elimination processes, and erection capability remain in good working order. My PSA remains at a static and safe sub 1.0 level during the entire period.

I am convinced at this point that selecting Dr. Peter Grimm, from the Seattle Prostate Institute, the best physician with that specialty in the world with the best equipment, was the right decision for my prostate oriented statistics and my physiological views. I've never felt better, nor savored life more, than I do right now. My improved eating habits have me at my college volleyball playing weight, 185 pounds vs. my previous of 192-195 pound level.

In retrospect, the only thing that would have made my road less pressured and the specific decision making process smoother would have been to have had immediate access to a book on prostate cancer like this one. Then, when first appraised by my HMO physician that I had flunked my prostate biopsy, I would have been prepared to deal with the dilemma with a great deal less stress and frustration. Doing the vigorous research also placed my mind in position to instruct my body that the right kind of help was on the way, leading to an affirmative result, which is the "Gold Medal" for these types of challenges.

All of my fellow case study suppliers and talented prostate cancer physicians have joined me by contributing their input for this specific purpose. I feel extremely strong about completing this compendium of special knowledge concerning this vital subject, and hope that it will present you with an early and important tool, both for preventative reasons, and for your sudden "need to know". Their contact information, along with my own, is supplied below, for any follow up questions that you may have. Good hunting, and please continue to stay informed!

COLLABORATOR MAILING LIST

ARCHER, Dick
1160 Fifee Lane
Santa Barbara, CA 93108
(805 969-0217)

BARRIOS, Al, PHD
11949 Jefferson Blvd.,
Culver City, CA 90230
(310 301-3317)

BENJAMIN, Harold, M.D.
2716 Ocean Park Blvd., Ste. 1040
Santa Monica, CA 90405-5211
(310 314-2555.2)

BROSMAN, Stanley, M.D.
1260 13th, Ste. 1200
Santa Monica, CA 90404
(310 458-4829)

FISHER, Stuart, M.D.
1260 15th St., Ste. 206
Santa Monica, CA 90404
(310 451-8751)

GRIMM, Peter, M.D.
1101 Madisson, Ste. 1101
Seattle, WA 98104
(800 422-4547x4)

MEYERS, Charles “Snuffy”, M.D.
(434 923-46460)

O'HARA, Michael
1239 El Hito Circle
Pacific Palisades, CA 90272

REGAN, Don
Newport Beach, CA
(949 280-1586)

ROSE, Chris, M.D.
501 S. Buena Vista
Burbank, CA 91505
(818 843-5111)

SCHOLZ, Mark, M.D.
LAM, Richard, M.D.
4676 Admiralty Way
Marina del Rey, CA 90292
(310 827-7707)

SHUMACHER, Jack
11693 San Vicente Blvd., Ste. 360
Los Angeles, CA 90049
(310 471-1280)

STEINBERG, Michael, M.D.
2428 Santa Monica Blvd., Ste. 103
Santa Monica, CA 90404
(310 828-0061)

TOOMEY, William
1755 High Mountain Road
Arroyo Grande, CA 93420
(805 481-6683)

WEINSTEIN, William K.
909 McGomery Street, Ste. 600
San Francisco, CA 94133
(415 677-1590)

ABOUT THE AUTHOR

Michael O'Hara's company, O'Hara Enterprises International, Inc. (OEI), has pioneered more college, professional and Olympic sporting endeavors than any company in history. OEI helped establish professional sports leagues in basketball, hockey and volleyball in the United States.

O'Hara has co-founded and co-owned teams that ultimately won a Stanley Cup and an NBA championship. O'Hara served as commissioner of two sports leagues as well as a college conference. One of the innovators of the three point play for basketball when helping form the American Basketball Association, O'Hara also conceived the Rally Scoring System for volleyball worldwide and was successful in initiating the addition of Beach Volleyball into the 1992 Olympic Games. He was one of two founders of the sport of Wallyball. His volleyball roles have included USVBA Board of Directors, U.S. representative to FIVB-Public Relations Committee and International Technical Director for Beach Volleyball.

O'Hara was vice-president of the Los Angeles Olympic Organizing Committee, responsible for the presentation of the 1984 Olympic Games. In addition to being the most successful single sporting event produced in the United States, the unique business approach established the legacy for all future Olympic Games.

Mr. O'Hara has served as a business instructor and volleyball coach at Santa Monica College over a 40 year period. He has been an expert commentator for all of the major networks. O'Hara has also completed assignments internationally including the first Good Will Games in 1988. He has also lectured worldwide on the topic of international sport, particularly the Olympic Games.

Athletically, O'Hara was a member of the United States Volleyball team that debuted the sport in the 1964 Olympic Games in Tokyo.

O'Hara with partner Mike Bright, won the first World Championships at Manhattan Beach, California. He is the only player in volleyball history worldwide, to be inducted into three Halls of Fame: Indoor Volleyball of Fame, YMCA Volleyball Hall of Fame and Beach Volleyball of Fame.